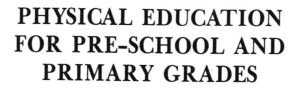

PHYSICAL EDUCATION
FOR PRE-SCHOOL AND
PRIMARY GRADES

Children's Letters To God

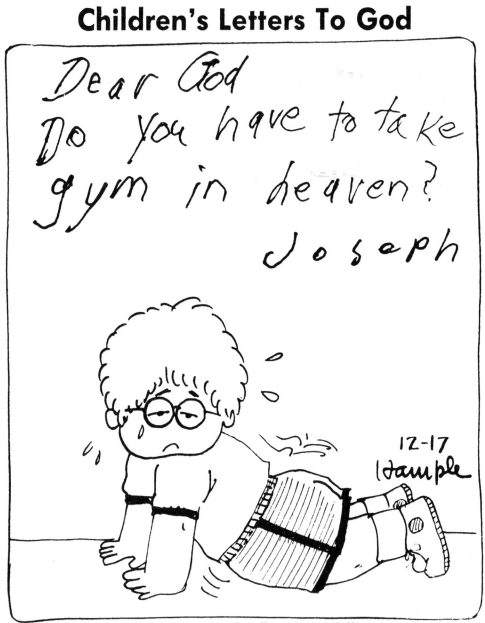

Second Edition

PHYSICAL EDUCATION FOR PRE-SCHOOL AND PRIMARY GRADES

By

NOELINE THOMPSON KELLY, ED.D.

and

BRIAN JOHN KELLY, PH.D.

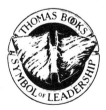

CHARLES C THOMAS • PUBLISHER, LTD.
Springfield • Illinois • U.S.A.

Published and Distributed Throughout the World by

CHARLES C THOMAS • PUBLISHER, LTD.
2600 South First Street
Springfield, Illinois 62794-9265

© *1997 by* CHARLES C THOMAS • PUBLISHER, LTD.

ISBN 0-398-06739-2 (paper)

Library of Congress Catalog Card Number: 96-40932

First Edition, 1985
Second Edition, 1997

Printed in the United States of America
SC-R-3

Library of Congress Cataloging-in-Publication Data

Kelly, Noeline Thompson.
    Physical education for pre-school and primary grades / by Noeline
Thompson Kelly, Brian John Kelly. — 2nd ed.
        p.   cm.
    Includes bibliographical references.
    ISBN 0-398-06739-2
    1. Physical education for children—Study and teaching.
2. Movement education.   3. Physical education for handicapped
children—Study and teaching.   4. Physical fitness for children.
I. Kelly, Brian John.   II. Title.
GV443.K455   1997
372.86′044—dc21   96-40932
                                                                        CIP

PREFACE

Current research has shown an alarming increase in obese children and a decline in their physical activity. This is not just a United States phenomenon, but is worldwide. Various reasons have been given for the decline in activity: changes in family lifestyles, single parent households, two parents working, limited play space, increased hours spent by children watching television and playing computer games, especially after school when parents are not home. Obesity in children has been attributed to poor nutritional habits, increased snacking, consumption of excessive calories of saturated fat and nonnutritious foods. Additionally, 25 percent of American children have blood cholesterol readings above an acceptable level. These childhood conditions may be predictors of heart disease and other health problems in adulthood.

Although most young American children are reasonably active, many obese children engage in minimal physical activity. It has become increasingly important for the pre-school caregiver and primary physical education teacher to compensate for the inactivity of children by providing *daily* activity time. Most physical education at the pre-school, kindergarten, and primary level is taught by caregivers and classroom teachers with minimal training in the area. They need a simple, sequential program guide for a full varied program. They need many ideas to cope with the short attention spans of young children. In most pre-school centers and elementary schools, activities take place outside in the playground with a minimal supply of equipment, and with children in street clothes. This text provides many activities for such conditions.

The teacher's attention is also drawn to the difference between *physical* fitness and *health-related* fitness. This text provides a novel, fun, physical fitness circuit instead of the traditional presentation.

It is recognized that the pre-school/primary level is the optimum learning period. Most simple movement patterns have already been established prior to entering school. It is time to define an activity program for that particular level, not just a watered down version of an intermediate level program (e.g., fitness circuits, calisthenics, kick ball).

The authors believe that a balance of all activities (time-wise) is necessary at the pre-school/primary level so that the interests of all children are accommodated and a strong foundation is established in the categories of games, dance, gymnastics, track and field, and, if at all possible, aquatics. These can all be introduced without playing up the competitive win-at-any-cost element.

Pre-school teachers of long-standing have noticed, over the years, changes in pre-school children's play. They report more passivity in pre-school children and an attitude, which the authors have also encountered, of "what is teacher going to do to entertain me today?" The span of attention of these children is limited and again puts pressure on teachers to organize activity periods which will, hopefully, retain pupil interest. A good teacher takes on the role of rehabilitator in motivating pre-school and primary grade children to become more active.

No one can seriously quarrel with either the need for play in its different forms, nor with the need for physical movement in the development of children. They do get better at movement as their movement experiences accumulate, and their capacity for physical response to their environments may be, in part, a function of the variability and richness of those experiences. Richness and variability in movement experiences may not arise from an environment that passively provides only equipment and play conditions. It is more likely to arise from situations consciously created to stimulate each child's movement potential, as a good teacher attempts to do.

Children deprived of the opportunity to achieve variability and range in movement activities may be compared with those children who watch television, or play computer games, to the exclusion of active play. Just as these children who are bereft of active play may lose the opportunity for the development of conceptual structures about themselves and their world, so may the inactive children never develop a generalized movement capacity on which to draw as they mature and interact with their environment and other children. Movement actions and manipulations of the self and others provide opportunity and practice in learning not only about the external environment but also about the child's own physical capabilities.

N.T.K.
B.J.K.

ACKNOWLEDGMENTS

The authors wish to give special recognition to Emilio Quieroz, illustrator; Kim Dennison-Moffat, Canada; John Barr, head teacher, Claremont Primary School, Alloa, Scotland; Joyce Ferguson, head teacher and Lesley Robertson, teacher, Abercromby Primary School, Alloa, Scotland; Keith Plunkett and John Sandos, New Zealand.

Special thanks are due the typists, Elsa Contreras and Maureen Brown.

CONTENTS

		Page
Preface		v
Chapter		
I.	ACTIVITIES TO STRETCH THE MUSCLES AND THE IMAGINATION	3
	Secret Bag	3
	Similes	5
	Changing Body Shapes	7
	Making Platforms For My Body	8
	Making Bridges With My Body	9
	Geometric Shapes	12
	Forming Letters, Names, and Numbers With My Body	13
	Words To Move To	15
	Boxes	16
	Hoops	17
	Tires	22
	Jump Ropes	25
	Stretch Ropes	27
	Scooters	31
	Kangaroo Bouncers	33
	Balance Boards	34
	Wands	34
	Parachute	35
	Ladder	38
II.	THROWING, CATCHING, AIMING, STRIKING ACTIVITIES, AND GAMES	40
	Progressions in Developing Sports Abilities	40
	Beanbags	42

Target Box 45
Clown Face 46
Wall Target 47
Wall Baskets 47
Bleach Bottle Catchers 48
Frisbees—Coffee Can Lids 49
Balls 50
Balloons, Beach Balls, Volleyballs 53
Plastic Baseball Bats and Tees 54
Goodminton 55
Mini Tennis 55
Rings 56
Handsie 57
Footsie 59
Juggling 59
Skittles 60
Relays: 60
    Tunnel Ball Relay 61
    Overhead Relay 61
    Bob Ball Relay 61
    Soccer Dribble Relay 62
Games: 62
    Keep the Basket Full 63
    All in Dodge Ball 63
    Knock the Tail Off 64
    Skittle Ball 64
    Jump the Beanbag 65
    Rotten Eggs 65
    Tee Ball 65
III. RACES, RELAYS AND CONTESTS 67
Mini Track and Field Meet Program 68
Novelty Races: 68
    Beanbag on Foot 68
    Piggies to Market 69
    Grocery Sack Race 69
    Shoebox Race 71

Car Race 71
Spider Ball 71
Push the Peanut 72
Kangaroo Race 72
Ball Under Chin 73
Skipping Rope 73
Siamese Twins 73
Ski Race 75
Novelty Relays: 75
Potato Relay 75
Egg and Spoon Relay 76
Chain Relay 77
Caterpillar Relay 77
Ball Through Hoops Relay 77
Obstacle Relay 78
In and Out Relay 78
Oxford Boat Race 79
City Gates Relay 79
Wheel Relay 79
Traditional Events: 80
Races 80
Relays 80
Jumps: 80
Standing Long Jump 80
Running Long Jump 81
Team Long Jump 81
High Jump (Scissors) 81
Vertical Jump 82
Hurdles 82
Throws 82
Contests: 82
Teepees 82
Jumping Circuit 82
Bridges 83
Dog and Bone 83
Lost Your Shadow 83

Center Ball Exchange 84
Beat Your Partner 84
Racing and Chasing Games: 84
    Tails 84
    Shadows 84
    What's the Time Mr. Wolf? 85
    Dry Feet, Wet Feet 85
    Daisy Chains 85
    Mr. Frost and Mrs. Thaw 86
    Cat and Mouse 86
    Fox and Geese 86
    Circle Chase 86
    Merry-Go-Round 87
    Shipwreck 87
    Streets and Lanes 87
IV.   BEGINNING TUMBLING AND GYMNASTICS 89
Gymnastics Fundamentals 90
Beginning Rolls: 91
    Hot Dog Roll 91
    Watermelon Roll 91
    Combination Rolls 91
    Egg Roll 92
    Shoulder Roll 92
    Forward Roll 92
        Forward Roll Variations 93
        Combination Rolls 94
    Backward Roll 94
        Rocking Chair 94
        Rock and Roll 94
        Backward Roll Variations 94
        Combination Rolls 94
Headstand 94
    Headstand Variations 95
    Combinations 97
Handstand 97
    Bunny Jump 97

Donkey Kick 97
Mule Kick 97
Handstand in Fours 97
Handstand in Twos 98
Handstand Variations 98
Combinations 98
Cartwheel 98
Combinations 98
Beginning Floor Exercise: 98
Floor Exercise Routines 99
Low Balance Beam 99
Horizontal Bar 102
Low Vaulting Box 104
Bench 105
Reuter Board: 106
Combinations 107
Long Hanging Ropes 107
V. DANCE ACTIVITIES 109
Dance Chart 110
Creative "Sow" Method Activities 111
Rhymes To Move To 111
Names To Move To 113
Creative Dance Using Rhythm Instruments 114
Creative Dance Using Patterns 118
Sounds To Move To 121
Verses and Poems 122
Dance a Story 125
Hats 126
Pictures Coming to Life 128
Statues 129
Sports 130
Shadows 131
Streamers and Scarves 132
Traditional "Show" Methods Activities 133
Icebreaker 133
Finger Plays 135

Action Songs: 136

    Bouncing Ball 136

    Digging 137

    Windmill 137

    Teapot 138

    Baby Ducks 138

Singing Games: 138

    Hammers 139

    Punchinello 141

    The Little Mice Are Creeping 142

    My Pigeon House 143

    The Thread Follows The Needle 144

    Alley, Alley, Oo 144

    A Tiny Little Woman 145

    Lubin Loo 145

    Market Gate 147

    I See a Tiny Little Cottage 148

Folk Dances: 149

    La Raspa (Mexico) 149

    Skip Annika (Sweden) 150

    La Vinca (Italy) 150

    Seven Jumps (Denmark) 151

    Clap Dance (Germany) 152

    Troika (Russia) 152

    Virginia Reel (America) 153

    Toast to King Gustav (Sweden) 154

    Square Dance (America) 154

Ethnic Dances: 156

    The Duck Dance (American Indian) 156

    Singing Up The Corn (American Indian) 156

    Dragon Dance (Indonesia) 158

    Poi Dance (New Zealand) 158

Jump Rope Rhymes 160

VI. FITNESS FOR LIFE 163

Shuttle Fun Run 165

Creepy Fingers 165

Long Jump Bump 165
Hot Feet Leap 166
Tarzan Ladder 166
Nosey Parker Peek 166
French Fry Fling 167
Fitness Circuit 168
Progress Charts 168
Positive Progress Report for Parents 169
VII.   WATER CONFIDENCE PLAY 173
Getting Into the Water: 174
  Humpty Dumpty 174
  Making Waves 174
  Follow the Leader 174
  Bouncing Ball 174
  Washing Machine 174
  Speedboats 174
  Whirlpool 174
  Elephants Bathing 174
  Birds Bathing 174
  Here, There, Where 174
  Seaplanes 176
  Crocodiles 176
  Balls 176
Getting Under the Water: 176
  Train Thru the Tunnel 176
  Circus Dog 176
  Polar Bear 176
  Frogs Catching Flies 176
  Seesaws 176
  Pop Goes the Weasel 176
  Jack in the Box 177
  Big A 177
  I Clap 177
  Submarines 178
  Turtles 178
Moving Through the Water: 178

Floating Bodies 178
Towing Logs 178
Gliding 178
Sculling 178

VIII.   PHYSICAL EDUCATION FOR SPECIAL POPULATIONS 179
Physical Education for the Disabled: 179
Mentally Retarded 181
Emotionally Disturbed 181
Learning Disabled 181
Orthopedically Handicapped 182
Visually Handicapped 182
Hearing Impaired 182
Speech Communication Impaired 183
Health Impaired 183
Seriously Obese 183
Crossing the Language Bridge in Physical Education . 184
Bilingual Education and Physical Education: 184
How to Present the Material 184
Basic Challenges Vocabulary 186
How to Build up a Challenge 186
Other Ways That the Two Languages Can Be Used
in Physical Education 186
Physical Education for the Gifted and Talented 187

IX.   METHODS OF TEACHING PHYSICAL EDUCATION 189
Planning a Physical Education Program: 189
Climate 189
Facilities and Surfaces 190
Equipment 191
Size of Class 191
Imagination of the Teacher 191
Program Pies 191
Lesson Plans 194
Methods: 196
"Show" Method 196
"Sow" Method 196
Basic Movements 197

How Do We Vary the Basic Movements? 198

Correlating Physical Education With Other Subjects . . 201

Teaching Hints: 202

    General 202

    Organization 202

    Spacing 203

    Moving 203

    Dividing 203

    Verbalizing 203

Assessment in Physical Education 204

Safety: 205

    Rules for a Safe Environment 205

    Prudent Teaching Strategies 205

    Supervision Strategies 206

    Safety First 206

    Wrongful Accusation 207

X.   PLAYGROUNDS AND EQUIPMENT 208

Essential Elements of a Playground 209

Equipment 211

Improvising Equipment 212

Wall Markings 225

Playground Markings 227

Appendices 229

Bibliography 235

PHYSICAL EDUCATION FOR PRE-SCHOOL AND PRIMARY GRADES

Chapter I

ACTIVITIES TO STRETCH THE MUSCLES AND THE IMAGINATION

In this chapter, the authors present activities that will not only exercise the body but will also call upon the children to exercise their minds, to let their imaginations take wings and to interpret the challenges presented in an original fashion. This may be a new approach to physical education, both for the teacher and the child. The authors believe that the readers will have few problems in teaching the activities presented if they follow the simple, laid-out organization steps and methodology. The challenges have been arranged from the simple to the more complex so that the teacher can proceed sequentially as each challenge is mastered.

SECRET BAG[1]

Objectives:

To draw original movement from the children using visual stimuli.
To exercise the body and imagination.

Equipment:

Large grocery bag.
Various objects, preferably moveable, in the bag.

Examples: a piece of elastic (stretch and contract), coffee can (roll and tilt), stapler, book, scissors, purse (open and shut), egg beater, rubber band, bottle (pop-off cork), clothes pin, silk scarf (wave and float in air), banana (peel it), ball (roll it, bounce it high and low, side to side, dribble it), tube of toothpaste (squeeze it), aerosol can (puff some out), salt shaker (tip and shake), ketchup bottle (tip up and hit bottom), teapot (pour it), floppy doll or animal (move the limbs, head, body calisthenics).

---

[1] Reprinted from *Instructor,* December, 1973. Copyright© 1973 by the Instructor Publications, Inc. Reprinted by permission of Scholastic, Inc.

Method:

Ask the children to sit or stand facing the bag of objects.

Reach into the bag and hold up an object so all the children can see it.

> *"Can you make yourself into this shape?...*
> *Now when I move it, see if you can move like it..."*

Return object to bag and bring out another one.

Wait until children have taken the shape before asking them to move like it.

Repeat several times, varying the type of object so that a variety of shapes and movements can be made.

At first the children tend to look around and copy each other.

Tell them to move any way they like, and praise the child with a different movement.

Do not demonstrate unless there is no response from the children.

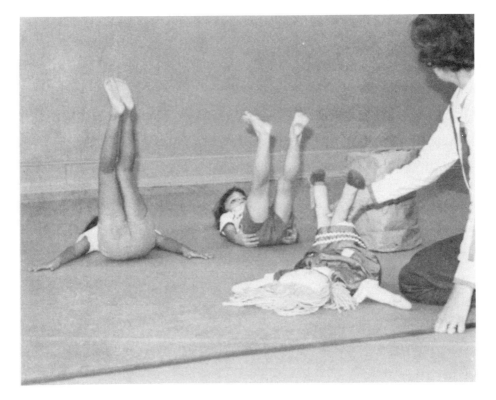

Figure 1. "Can you move your legs like the doll?"

SIMILES

Objectives:

To draw original movement from the children.
To exercise the body and imagination.

Method:

(Note: There are two kinds of similes: (1) single-barreled simile—fly like a pigeon; and (2) double-barreled simile—fly like a pigeon that has eaten too much.)
The latter type draws a more original and complex interpretation from the child.
Ask the children to find their very own space so that they can see you, you can see them, and they have room to move.
Use similes that are within their range of experience. Choose from the list supplied or make up your own. Notice the wide variety of body movements involved in the similes below.
Call out the similes in an expressive manner.
Give the children time to experiment with the challenge you have given them.
Move around the class praising them.
At first they will tend to copy each other.
Do not demonstrate unless there is no response from the children.
Give the next simile.
Try to alternate a vigorous locomotor simile with one performed on the spot.

Examples: Wobble like Jello™ on a plate.
Jump like a pogo stick in the mud.
Walk like a baby learning to walk.
Hop like a hammer has been dropped on your toe.
Skip like a giant with big boots.
Stretch like a puppy waking from a nap.
Move like air bubbles in a fish tank.
Crawl like a tired caterpillar.
Pop like a bursting soap bubble.
Move like lips when someone is talking.
Float upward like a balloon—pop!
Walk like a giraffe with a very stiff neck.

Roll like toothpaste coming out of the tube.
Crawl like an ant carrying a big crumb.
Wiggle like a worm on the hot ground.

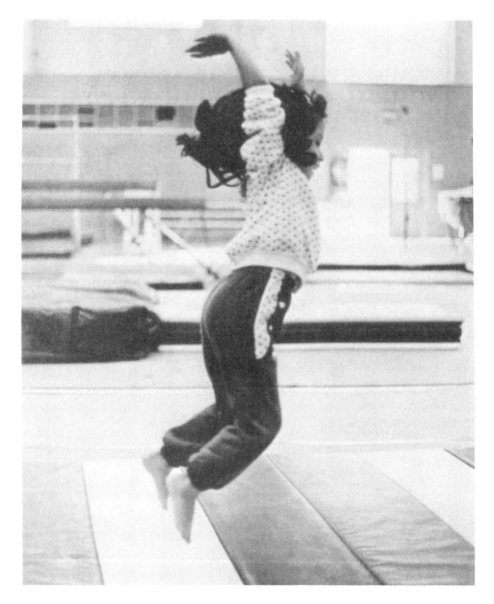

Figure 2. "Jump like a teenager."

Jump like cheerleaders who have won a game.
Wiggle like a bug that mother has sprayed.
Shake like a dog that has just been washed.
Walk as if you have chewing gum stuck to your shoe.
Fly like Superman.
Swim like a goldfish in a bowl that is too small.
Roll like a pop can over a bumpy sidewalk.
Open like a flower under a sprinkler.
Melt like an ice cube in the sun.
Walk like an elephant who has eaten too many peanuts.
Move like a garbage truck coming down your alley.
Move like you are just learning to roller skate.
Move like a wheelbarrow with a heavy load.
Move your legs like a pair of scissors.

CHANGING BODY SHAPES

Objectives:

To stimulate the children's perception and awareness of different shapes
   by forming them with their bodies.
To exercise the body and imagination.

Method:

Ask the children to find their very own space so they can see you, you
   can see them, and they have room to move.
Give them verbal challenges, such as:

> *"Show me how you can make your body into the shape of a banana...*
> *Now show me how you can make your body into the shape of a grape...*
> *And now let me see you take the shape of a watermelon..."*
> (Note the three contrasts in shape and size.)

> *"Now when I call out the names of those fruits, I want you to change your*
> *body into those shapes...*

> *Banana...grape...watermelon...banana...watermelon...grape...*
> *banana..."*

Give the children time to take each shape; gradually quicken up words so
   children quicken up changes.
Do not demonstrate unless there is no response from the children.
Move around the class praising original shapes.

Use the names of other vegetables, fruits, objects, as verbal cues, aiming
for contrast between shapes.

Examples: Leaf, flower, tree.
Table, window, chair.
Cup, coffee pot, plate.
Soap, toothbrush, toothpaste.
Comb, hairbrush, mirror.
Hamburger, french fry, drinking straw.
Snake, giraffe, tiger.

MAKING PLATFORMS FOR MY BODY

(Changing Bases of Support)

Objectives:

To increase the children's awareness of body parts.
To develop balance.
To increase efficiency in transferring body weight to different body
parts.
To exercise the body and imagination.

Method:

Ask the children to find their very own space so they can see you, you
can see them, and they have room to move.
Give them verbal challenges such as those listed below.
Move around the class, praising and encouraging original movements.
Do not demonstrate unless there is no response from the children.

> *"Let me see you balance on one part of your body...*
> *That is your platform...*
>
> *Now can you balance on another part of your body?...*
> *That is another platform...*
>
> *Now when I say 'change,' go back to your first platform... 'change!'*
> *Now when I say 'change,' keep changing from one platform to the other...*
> *'change'... 'change'..."*

(Speak slowly to start and then get faster.)

A progression from the above activity is to ask the children to choose three different platforms and to number them 1, 2, and 3.

When the teacher calls out a number, the children change to the appropriate platform.

Changes can be done slowly or fast.

Another approach to the above activity is to ask the children to stand, sit, kneel, or lie on the ground and to feel what is touching the ground.

Tell them that whatever is touching the ground is their "platform."

Ask them to move their bodies so that another part is touching the ground.

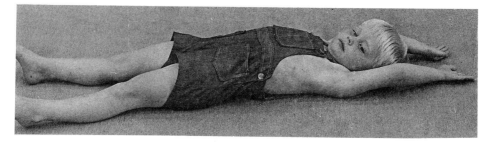

Figure 3. "Whatever is touching the ground is your platform."

Then they can change back and forth between these two platforms.

A third approach is to ask the children to find as many different platforms for their bodies as they can.

Let half the class at a time show the other half what they can do.

MAKING BRIDGES WITH MY BODY

Objectives:

To increase flexibility and balance.

To develop muscles and support body weight.

To exercise the body and imagination.

Method:

Ask the children to find their very own space so they can see you, you can see them, and they have room to move.

Closed challenge (one in which you can anticipate the type of response):

1. *"Can you make a bridge with your body keeping two hands and two feet on the ground?...*

Now can you make it very high?...

Now can you make it very low?...

Let me see your bridge go from very low to very high, and back to very low, moving slowly and carefully ... rest ...

Now let me see your bridge get very wide, then very narrow, very wide again, then very narrow again ... rest ...

This time let me see your bridge get very high and very narrow; now very low and very wide ... (repeat)

2. *"Can you make a bridge with your body keeping two hands and one foot on the ground? ..."*

Add variations similar to number 1.

3. *"Can you make a bridge using just one hand and one foot?...*

"Now can you use the other hand and foot?...

When you hear me say 'change,' use the other hand and foot ... 'change' ... 'change' ... 'change' ..."

Add variations similar to number 1.

Open challenge (one which gives the children a chance to be more imaginative):

"Can you make a bridge with your body?
You can do it any way you like ..."

Look around the class and notice the different interpretations.

"Let us look at the different bridges you have made ...
John, will you show us your bridge? ... very good ...
Let's all do John's bridge ...
Now, Mimi, will you show us your bridge? ...
Let's all do Mimi's bridge ..."

Repeat for several different children, praising constantly.
Add variations to the children's bridges; higher, lower, wobbly, etc.

"Now can you make a bridge that no one else has made before? ..."

Let several children show their bridges for the others to copy.

With Partner (this increases the creative possibilities):

> *"Can you make a bridge that opens to let big ships pass through?...*
> *Open your bridge ... close your bridge ... open ... close ...*
> *Can you make a bridge with a high tower at each end?...*
>
> *Let me see a low, wide bridge with a flag waving on a tall pole ...*
>
> *Show me a narrow, rickety bridge with a hole in the middle ...*
>
> *Can one of you make a little bridge and the other be the water flowing under it?... "*

In Threes or Fours:

> *"Let me see you make a bridge that has high arches ...*
> *Can you now put two flagpoles on it?...*
> *And now can you show it to me shaking in the wind?...*
>
> *Can you make a narrow swinging bridge?...*
> *Make it swing gently as if someone is crossing it ...*
>
> *Now make me a busy bridge with lots of cars crossing it.*
> *It will have to be strong!... "*

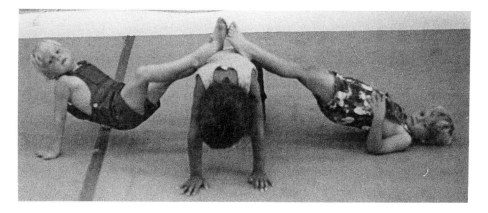

Figure 4. "Make a bridge with high arches."

Add variations similar to previous challenges.
Let groups show the class their efforts.

GEOMETRIC SHAPES

Objectives:

To increase awareness of different geometric shapes, sizes, and colors.
To increase agility.

Equipment:

Wooden geometric shapes, square, rectangle, triangle, circle, diamond,
 oval, octagon; large and small sizes, painted in different colors.
Supports to keep shapes upright.
These can be constructed (see "Improvising Equipment" in Chapter X).
Foam shapes and standards are available commercially.
Small mats, beanbags, balls.

Method:

This activity is best done by a small group while the rest of the class has
 another activity.
Stand shapes, in supports, in a random formation.
Use mats if surface is rough.

> *"Let me see you creep through the shapes and tell me their names...*
> *Now as you creep through, tell me what color they are...*
> *This time crawl through a big red triangle and run around a little blue
> square..."*

Repeat, using different locomotor movements, including spider walk,
 crab walk, bunny jump.
Introduce different colors, shapes, and sizes.
Place shapes flat on the ground.

> *"Everyone stand beside a shape...*
> *Let me see you make your body into that shape and tell me its name...*
> *Now run to another shape and do the same thing..."*

Repeat several times, using hop, jump, skip, gallop, slide.
Use shapes for prepositional challenges.

> *"Everyone stand beside a shape and tell me its name...*
> *What color is it?...*
> *Show me how nicely you can jump in and out of it...*
> *Jump up and down inside it...*

Hop in and out...
Leap over...
Skip around...
Walk feet around it like a compass...
Spider walk around it...
Balance on one foot and one hand in it...
Balance on two hands and one foot in it...
Make a bridge across it, tummy facing the sky... now tummy facing the
   ground..."

For additional challenges, see "Hoops" in this chapter.

With Partner:

Teacher holds up shape, asks children to make that shape with their
   partners.
Draw attention to different interpretations, upright, and on the ground.
Children toss beanbags or balls to each other through the shapes, nam-
   ing them and their colors.

In Groups:

Use in obstacle relays to creep through, run around, toss a beanbag
   through, leap across.
Play "Follow the Leader," doing whatever and going wherever the leader
   goes.

FORMING LETTERS, NAMES, AND NUMBERS
WITH MY BODY

Objectives:

To recognize letters, sounds, names, and numbers.
To develop number symbols sense.
To increase flexibility and balance.
To transform symbols into body shapes.
To encourage cooperation.

Equipment:

Blackboard, chalk, eraser, large signs, letters, numbers.

Method:

Free spacing, facing teacher and blackboard or wall.

Write letters, numbers, or names of people and objects on blackboard or
hold up signs.

> *"Who knows the name of this letter?...*
> *What sound does it make?...*
> *Let me see you make that letter with your body..."*

Some children will respond with shapes while standing up, others will
form them on the ground, others against the wall.

Move around the class praising their efforts.

Repeat with other letters.

> *"I am writing two letters on the board.*
> *They are the beginning letters of someone's names.*
> *Whose are they?... That's right, Brian.*
> *They belong to you. Brian begins with a B, and Jones begins with a J.*
> *Let me see you make Brian's letters with your partner.*
> *You can lie on the ground to do this..."*

In Threes, Fours, Fives, etc.:

> *"Today I am writing someone's name on the board.*
> *Who owns this name?... That's right, Amy.*
> *It is your name.*
> *How many children will you need to make your name?...*
> *That's right, three.*
> *Let me see you all get into groups of three and make Amy's name..."*

Move around class helping children to group.

Repeat, using another child's name with three letters.

Gradually use longer names involving larger group cooperation.

Forming Numbers:

Start with children working on their own.

Write number "2" on blackboard.

> *"Who knows what this number is?...*
> *That's right, James, It is the number '2.'*
> *Can you all show me two fingers?... two eyes... two ears... two heads... two*
> *   boys... two girls...*
> *Now when I say '2,' let me see you run and hold hands in 2's.*

Ready!... '2'!!... Good!...
Now let me see those 2's jump up and down like bouncing balls... "

Give other pair activities such as "Wash the dishes," "See Saw," "Teepees," "Push Me, Pull You."

Repeat, using 3, 4, etc., getting children to form groups, and do an action while in the group.

Adding and subtracting can be introduced by having children joining or leaving a group.

WORDS TO MOVE TO

Objectives:

To stimulate original interpretation.
To develop vocabulary and knowledge of word meanings.
To exercise the whole body.

Method:

Teacher makes a list of action words which lend themselves to interpretation in movement.

"Today I'm going to say some words which tell you how to move...
Find your very own space and, when you move, try not to bump into anyone... "

Teacher says a familiar word such as walk (jump, hop) to see if the children understand what she means them to do.

Then she introduces less familiar words such as spin, float, prance.

Then the words are combined into sequences such as float, spin, fall, and wiggle, stretch, wobble.

The following are action words that could be used:

Fly, sink, roll, crouch, pounce, scratch, slither, creep, curl up, rock, shiver, twist, turn, climb.

This is a good time to use similes.

Teacher then introduces emotional words and asks the children to move as if they are happy, sad, etc.

The following are emotional words:

Surprised, scary, curious, frightened, hurt, nervous, excited, tired, thirsty, lost (and then found), lazy, sick, ticklish, itchy, squashed, punished, bored, sleepy.

"Show me how you would move if you were very tired...
Now let's all move as if we are very nervous...
This time show me that you are very ticklish..."

BOXES[2]

(Prepositional Challenges)

Objectives:

To introduce prepositions in an informal and concrete way.
To increase awareness of direction.
To increase cardiovascular efficiency.
To exercise the whole body.
To increase efficiency in locomotor movements.
To distinguish between the "hop" and the "jump."

Equipment:

Cardboard boxes (from the supermarket) with tops removed: some very
   low, some apple-box size, depending on the size of the children; one
   for each child.
Hoops, short ropes, plastic crates or balls could also be used.

Method:

Free spacing, standing beside boxes, facing teacher.
Emphasize the prepositions with voice.

"Can you walk around your box without touching it?...
Now run around your box...
Can you skip around your box?...
Now can you walk backwards around it?
Look over your shoulder...
Show me how you can jump into your box...
Now jump out of it... in again... out... in...
Let me see you jump up and down in your box...
Now jump out and stand way back from it...
Show me how you can leap across your box...

---

[2]Reprinted from *Instructor,* October 1973. Copyright© 1973 by the Instructor Publications, Inc. Reprinted
by permission of Scholastic, Inc.

Use your arms to help you go higher...
Do it again and again... try to leap higher!...
Let's all leap across five boxes and then rest...
Try not to bump into anyone...
Now lie beside your box and then roll away from it...
Now roll towards your box... roll away... roll back...
This time let me see you crawl under your box and keep very still...
Now can you move along the ground, keeping under your box?... "

Choose different interpretations for the other children to copy.

"Now stand behind your box and see if you can hop on one foot into it
... hop out... hop in...
Use your other foot this time... "

This is a good time to distinguish between the "hop—a one-to-one foot movement—and the "jump"—a two-foot landing.
Tell the children to place their boxes at the side of the play area.
Take one large box and ask them to take the shape of it.

"Now, as I move this box, you move just like it... "

Tilt the box forward, backwards and sideways, rock it, lay it on its side, stand it on its end, turn it over and over sideways, so that the children roll to the side of the play areas and finish in a wriggling pile.
This is a good time to introduce beanbag or ball throwing into the boxes (see "Beanbags" and "Balls" in Chapter II.)

HOOPS[3]

Objectives:

To increase cardiovascular efficiency, agility, coordination and dexterity.
To elicit original movements.
To provide prepositional challenges.

Equipment:

Plastic hoops of various sizes; one for each child.
These can be made cheaply (see "Improvising Equipment" in Chapter X).

---

[3]Reprinted from *Instructor,* March 1974. Copyright© 1974 by the Instructor Publications, Inc. Reprinted by permission of Scholastic, Inc.

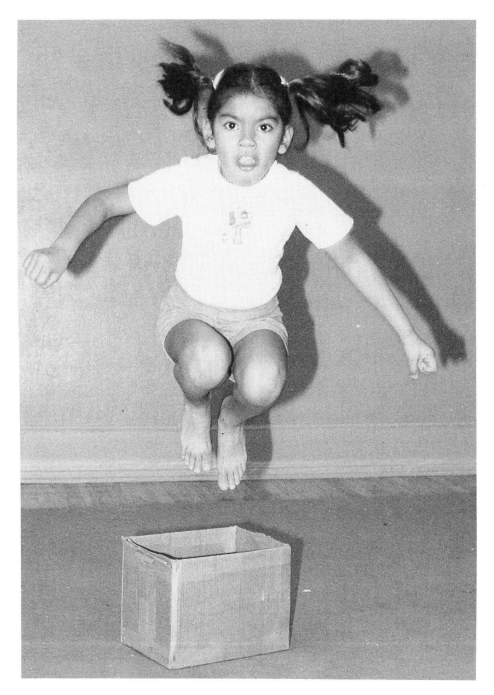

Figure 5. "Show me how you can jump over your box."

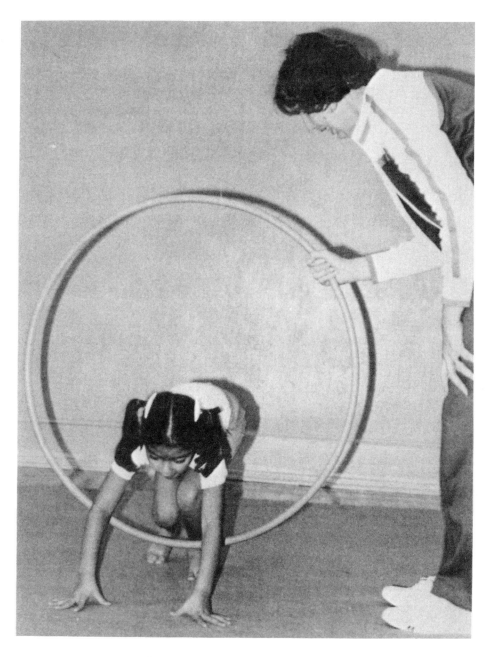

Figure 6. "Bunny jump through the hoop."

Method:

Free spacing, facing teacher.

Informal Approach

Define boundaries of play area and let children play freely with their
  hoops for about three minutes.

Do not allow huluing around the neck because of possible injury from
  loose staples or rough inner surfaces.

Most children will try to hulu the hoop around the waist.

Praise different moves such as bowling, spinning, skipping.

Let children show what they have been doing for class to copy.

Formal Approach

"Put your hoop on the ground and let me see you walk around it . . . "

Repeat, using run, hop, jump, skip, gallop, slide.

"Pretend your hoop is a puddle of water . . .
Let me see you jump into your puddle with a big splash . . . step out, and do
  it again . . .
Now stay in your puddle and swim around like a duck . . .
Now pretend that your hoop is a tightrope at the circus . . .

Let me see you walk around it without falling off . . . now sideways . . . now
  using your hands and feet like a monkey . . .

Let's pretend that your hoops are stepping stones across a lake . . .
Put them close enough to each other so that you can get from one to
  another without getting your feet wet . . .
Now let me see you step across to another hoop . . . and another . . . and
  another . . . "

Repeat, using jump, hop, leap.

"Now let's pretend that your hoop is a bunny hole.
Show me that you can bunny jump in and out of your hole . . . "

Repeat, using around, across.

"Sit on the ground and pretend that your hoop is a big hat . . .
Raise your hat . . . lower it . . . tilt it to the side . . . now to the other side.
Pretend your hoop is an angel's halo.
Stretch it high above your head . . . lower it . . .
Now hold your hoop in front of you like a big mirror . . .
Show me a happy face . . . sad . . . pretty . . . ugly . . . scary . . . etc.

> *Let's all stand up and show me how you can hulu the hoop around your waist . . .*
> *Start it up high under your armpits . . .*
> *Can you still hulu while you walk forward? . . . backwards? . . . sideways? . . .*
> *Can you make the hoop hulu around your knees? . . . "*

Repeat, using ankles, one leg as in "Footsie," one arm or wrist.

> *"Spread out and see if you can toss your hoop in the air and catch it . . .*
> *Now let me see you use your hoop like a jump rope to skip . . . "*

Repeat, turning hoop forward, backwards; moving forward, backwards; swinging hoop sideways under feet. "Bluebells" and then overhead.
Have children line up across play area.

> *"Let me see you bowl your hoop across the playground and run beside it . . .*
> *This time bowl it hard and chase it . . .*
> *Now bowl it and see if you can race it to the line . . . "*

Repeat, using run around, run through.

With Partner:

One child holds hoop low and horizontal, while partner steps into and out of it.
Repeat, using jump, hop into, crawl, creep under and out of.
One child holds hoop low and vertical, while partner creeps, runs, or bunny jumps through.
One child spins hoop, while partner imitates its movement with his/her body.
One child bowls hoop past partner, who tries to run through it.
Children bowl hoop back and forth to each other.

In Groups:

Teacher or children hold hoops vertically one yard apart to form a tunnel.
Other children line up at end of tunnel and bunny jump, creep, or run low through the hoops.
Play "In the Pond, Out of the Pond."
Children put their hoops on the ground and stand behind them.
Teacher calls out "In the pond . . . Out of the pond . . . In the pond . . . Out of the pond."

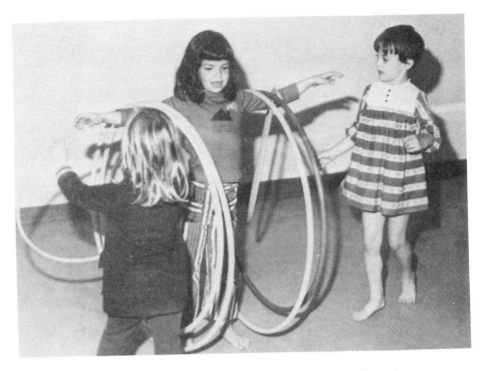

Figure 7. "Hang your hoops on Heather's arms."

Children jump in and out of their hoops.

If they jump or (later) move in the wrong direction, they must sit in their pond.

The last children standing are the winners.

Do not allow game to go on too long to avoid children sitting still.

Change the command to "In . . . Out . . . In . . . Out" to quicken reactions.

Hoops can be collected at the end of the lesson by having children stand with arms flexed sideways for hoops to be hung on them.

Or, have two children stand facing away from class with faces covered, while others stand up closely and "hoopla" the hoops over their bodies.

TIRES

Objectives:

To develop muscular strength and endurance, balance, agility, and coordination.

To increase accuracy in aiming.

Equipment:

Tires—from autos, airplanes, tractors, bicycles.

Inner tubes, beanbags, balls.

Wash tires, drill holes for drainage, check for spiders, etc., each time before using.

Method:

Informal Approach

Free play with tires in designated area.

Draw attention to different activities.

Let the other children copy.

Formal Approach

Have children place tires on ground.

Use like hoops for prepositional challenges.

> *"Let me see you jump in and out of your tire . . .*
> *Now step across from one side to the other . . .*
> *Now balance on one leg . . . try not to fall off . . .*
> *Can you jump right over your tire? . . .*
> *Can you walk around on it sideways? . . . "*

Repeat, using forward, backwards.

> *"Let's all do jumping jacks in and out of our tires . . .*
> *Now show me you can bunny jump in and out . . .*
> *Put your hands inside your tire and walk your feet all the way around outside like a compass . . .*
> *Can you spider walk, with tummy up, all the way around? . . .*
> *Keep your hands in the center . . . "*

Repeat, using tummy down.

Place tires in zigzag formation.

Have children walk and run over them, jump from one to the other, spider walk over them.

> *"Now let's all line up at the side of the play area and bowl our tires to the other side . . .*
> *Try to keep up with your tire and push it on the top with your hand . . . "*

Repeat, using run beside it, behind it, in front of it, race it to the line, fall down when it falls down.

Aim tire to knock down a milk carton or to pass between two cones.
Throw beanbags into tire on the ground.
Throw beanbags or balls through tire suspended on a rope.
Crawl through, or climb over, tire set into the ground.

With Partner:

> *"Can you walk your hands around the tire while your partner holds your*
>   *legs? (wheelbarrow position)...*
> *Can you do pushups in this position?...*
> *Let's all have a tug of war with our partners...*
> *Try to pull him/her over the line...*
> *Now show me that you can bowl the tire to your partner without it*
>   *wobbling..."*

Repeat several times; add trying to hit a milk carton in the middle.
Suspend tires on ropes.
Have children toss beanbags or balls through them.
Then record the number of good tosses.
See who has the highest.

In Groups:

Use many of the above activities in relay races.
Do not have more than six in a team.
Use tires in an obstacle course.
Bowl one tire, crawl through the next, walk with the next one around
    waist, leap across the next, zigzag run over the next tires, throw
    beanbag through the suspended tire.
Play "In the Pond, Out of the Pond" (see "Hoops" in this chapter).
Suspend tires on chains to form swings.
Build a climbing frame (see "Improvising Equipment" in Chapter X).
Use tractor tires to make a sand pit.
Use large inner tube to make a mini tramp (see "Improvising Equipment"
    in Chapter X).
Use bicycle inner tubes for tug of war, chest expanders, stretch rope
    activities, tails.

JUMP ROPES

Objectives:

To increase cardiovascular efficiency, flexibility, agility, and coordination.
To encourage original movement.

Equipment:

Short ropes of different lengths (use window sash cord), one for each
child.
Rope should stretch from armpit to armpit when child is standing on the
midline.
Make sure ropes are the correct length for each child.
Wind surplus rope around hands.
Use long sash cord ropes for group activities.

Method:

Free spacing in designated area.

Informal Approach
Let children experiment with ropes.
Look around the class to choose different activities for the children to
copy.
Develop the lesson from the children's ideas.

Formal Approach
(Note: Learning to jump rope can be frustrating.)
Children learn best by copying their classmates, rather than by teacher
breaking down the movement.

> *"Today we are going to try to jump rope like Janie...*
> *Watch her jump rope and see if you can do it, too..."*

Move around the class praising efforts, giving verbal cues, adjusting
rope length.
As the simple 2 to 2 foot jump, with and without a rebound, is achieved,
add the following progressions:
Move forward, backwards, sideways.
Turn rope backwards, cross arms.
Jump high, low (squat).
Hop, with and without rebound; alternate feet.
Leap forward over rope, turning rope high.

Point toe forward while hopping; tap toe forward.

Two jumps with rebound, twirl rope to left and right of body.

Twirl rope in Figure 8, then twirl rope overhead like a lariat.

Fold rope, hold both ends in one hand, twirl rope in a low circle and jump over it.

Twirl overhead, then under feet.

Repeat, moving forward.

Use as a barrier on the ground for prepositional challenges (see "Stretch Ropes" in this chapter).

Manipulate with bare feet.

Grip with toes, lift leg forward, sideways, backwards.

Make shapes on ground: geometric, animal, flower, number, name (group effort).

Sit on ground, grip rope with toes, roll backwards and pass overhead, return to sit.

With Partner:

One child twirls rope in a circle while other child jumps over it.

One child jumps rope while other child runs in to jump same rope; facing partner, back to partner, behind partner.

Partners stand side by side, each holding an end of the rope, jump rope on the spot, then moving forward.

Play "Horse and Driver." One child hooks rope around waist and gallops around, while driver gallops behind, holding the reins.

In Threes:

Two children turn rope while other child jumps in the middle.

Repeat, adding, move forward, backwards, hops, straddle jumps, hot peppers (fast jumps), jumps over rope raised higher off the ground, "High Water"; jumps over rope swinging back and forth, but not over head, "Bluebells"; low squat jumps, "Ducks."

Two children kneel, hold rope loosely to form a hurdle, other child leaps over as if hurdling, then bunny jumps and cartwheels.

Using Long Ropes:

Most activities for short ropes can be adapted for long ropes.

Change rope holders frequently.

Start with "Bluebells" to develop timing before turning rope overhead.

Have children stand beside rope, then add: *"run in, jump, run out, run through, follow the leader, doing whatever (s)he does."*

Play "Snakes and Ladders" in which the rope is wriggled from side to side, on the ground (snakes), and undulated up and down (ladders), while children leap across, and try not to touch it.

Play "Jump the Shot." One child twirls a rope with a tennis ball or beanbag tied on the end while other children jump it.

Rope must be kept close to ground.

Change twirler frequently to avoid dizziness.

STRETCH ROPES

Objectives:

To increase awareness of shapes, size, height, width, distance, etc.
To learn the names of geometrical shapes.
To exercise the whole body and increase cardiovascular efficiency.
To increase accuracy in throwing and catching.

Equipment:

Short circular stretch ropes (Chinese jump ropes), or pieces of elastic stitched firmly to form a loop, or rubber bands looped together.
One rope for each child.
Large geometrical shapes on cardboard or drawn on a blackboard.
Long stretch ropes (German or magic), at least one for every ten children.

Method:

Using short ropes, free spacing, facing the teacher.

> *"Put your foot down on the end of your rope . . .*
> *See how high you can stretch it . . . how low can it go? . . .* (repeat)
> *Now show me how wide you can stretch your rope . . .*
> *How narrow? . . . "* (repeat)

Show the class a square.

> *"Who knows the name of this shape? . . . That's right, it is a square.*
> *How many sides does it have?*
> *What do you notice about the sides? . . .*
> *They are all the same size.*
> *How many corners does it have?*

Who knows what those corners are called?...
That's right! They are called angles...
Can you make a square with your rope?
You will have to use your hands and feet to help you... "

Some children will make the shape standing up; others will do it on the
   ground.
Draw attention to the different interpretations.
Show the class a rectangle.
Draw attention to the two long sides and the two short sides.

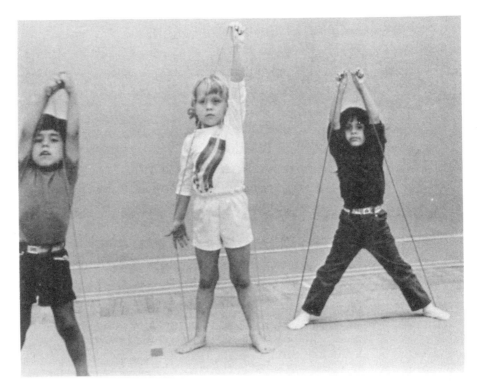

Figure 8. "Can you make a triangle with your rope?"

Use the same approach as for the square.
Repeat, with triangle, circle, diamond, star, flower, animal, fruit, window,
   etc.
Ropes can be placed on the ground and used for locomotor activities
   such as puddles to jump over, stepping stones, bunny holes, tightrope
   walk (see "Hoops" in this chapter).

With Partner (sharing one rope):

> *"Can you make a square with your rope, and can your partner make a square with his/her body?..."*

Repeat, using other shapes, alternating the child using the rope.

> *"Can you and your partner make a square with your rope?..."*

Repeat, using other shapes, and introducing tall, short, fat, thin, wide, narrow, small, huge, etc.

Have one child put the rope around his/her waist to become a horse, and the other child hold the loop like reins, to become the driver.

> *"Let me see you gallop around the playground without bumping into anyone...*
>
> *Pretend you have to jump over fences (or logs) on the way..."*

Alternate horse and driver.

In Threes (sharing one rope):

> *"Let me see two of you make your rope into a window like this* (show a vertical rectangle)...
>
> *Now let me see your friend step through it without touching it..."*

Repeat using creep, jump, hop, bunny jump.
Alternate children frequently.

> *"Let me see you make a trap door like this..."*
> (show a low, horizontal rectangle)

Repeat above movements.

In Fours (sharing one rope):

Have two children make a high, vertical window (rectangle).
Other two children toss beanbag or ball through it, trying not to touch the sides.
Count how many successful tosses.
Decrease size of window.
Increase distance from window.
Change rope holders frequently.

Using Long Stretch Ropes:

(Note: Take care that the child holding the rope loops the end around his/her wrist and also grasps the rope with two hands. Or, additionally, place rope around the waist before looping wrist and grasping rope.)

Stretch as many ropes as available across the play area.
Have children line up in team formation, facing ropes.

> *"Let me see the first row run and leap over the ropes . . . "*

Repeat with each row.

> *"This time let us leap over the first rope and crawl under the next . . . "*

Repeat, using jump, hop, gallop, creep, etc.
Raise or lower the ropes.
Change rope holders frequently.
Hold ropes high.
Have children bounce up to touch rope with their heads.
Volley balloons or balls over ropes.
Hold ropes low.
Have children line up at end of rope and bunny jump along from side to side.
Maintain good spacing between children.
(Note: This rope can also be used when teaching the cartwheel to get legs stretched higher.)
Tie rope into a circle and place on the ground.
Have children sit inside rope and try to lift it with their feet over their heads, into the circle, and back again. This is best done with bare feet.
Have children sit outside rope and grasp it.
Try to draw knees to chest and stretch legs over rope to center.
Reverse this movement . . . (repeat several times).
Use the rope circle as a tightrope to walk around without stepping off, walk backwards, sideways, high on toes, low with bent knees (duck), on all fours (monkey).
Sideways jump and hop in and out of circle, on the spot, moving forward, backwards.
Play "In the Pond, Out of the Pond" (see "Hoops" in this chapter).

In Groups:

Have two children make a high, wide, vertical rectangle.
Other children throw beanbags or balls back and forth through the window.
Make window narrower by stretching the rope wider.
Have two children make a low, horizontal rectangle.

Other children step into and out of it.

Repeat, using jump, leap, hop, scissor high jump, into the rectangle; then crawl, creep, and roll out of the rectangle.

SCOOTERS

Objectives:

To develop muscular strength, particularly in the upper body and legs.

To increase awareness of direction and space.

To increase steering ability.

To stimulate the imagination.

Equipment:

Scooters, 16″ × 16″, enough for one group to use while the rest of class engage in other activities.

These are easily constructed.

Moulded plastic scooters with handles are available commercially.

Milk cartons or cone markers, with tops cut flat, to support a wooden dowel.

Beanbags, jump ropes.

Tape or chalk to make traffic lanes or use playground markings.

Method:

(Note: Never allow children to stand on scooters.)

Establish traffic lanes.

Encourage children to look over shoulders when moving backwards.

Maintain wide spacing between children.

> *"Let me see you lie on your tummy (or middle),*
> *stretch your legs, and use your hands to move forward...*
> *Follow the line and don't bump into anyone..."*

There will be two interpretations: hands moving together or alternately.

Encourage children to try both ways.

Repeat, moving backwards, follow-the-leader, in zigzags, curves, circles, around cone markers or milk cartons, under mats shaped into tents, under hurdles made with cones and wands, slowly twirling on the spot like a helicopter.

The following activities must be done with all children moving in the same direction and widely spaced.

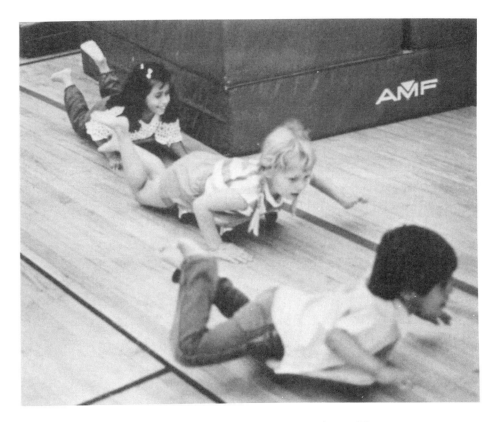

Figure 9. "Use your hands to move forward."

"Now move like a crocodile, through the mud, looking for his dinner . . .
This time pretend you are on a surfboard . . .
Paddle slowly . . . here comes a big wave . . .
Paddle to shore as hard as you can! . . .
Now sit on your scooter and push yourself along with your feet . . .
look over your shoulder . . .
Now tuck your feet up and push with your hands . . .
forward and backwards . . .
This time, kneel on your scooter and use your hands to move forward . . . "

Repeat above movements.

"Now kneel on one knee and scoot yourself along with your other foot.
Watch out for other children . . . "

With Partner:

Join up one behind the other, front child sits with feet tucked up, back
child sits with feet on front scooter.

Use hands to move forward.

Repeat above movements.

Line up opposite partner, move towards each other and exchange beanbag while passing.

Pull partner along with rope, not too fast!

Children lie on scooters, back child holds ankles of front child and
pushes with toes, and front child uses hands to move pair forward.

In Groups:

Make a train by having children sit on scooters, place feet on scooter in
front of them, and push with their hands to move forward.

Encourage children to work together to keep joined up.

Take the same formation, but pretend children are in a canoe, using
alternate hands to move forward.

KANGAROO BOUNCERS

Objectives:

To develop total body coordination.
To develop leg strength.

Equipment:

Large inflatable balls with loops on top.

Method:

Establish traffic lanes.
Maintain wide spacing between children.

> *"Sit on your ball, hold on to the loop,*
> *gently bounce up and down...*
> *Now try to jump forward...*
> *Can you jump on your ball and turn around?..."*

Have children form a line and play Follow The Leader.
Have children form a circle and jump forward.

BALANCE BOARDS

Objectives:

To develop balance and coordination.
To develop accuracy in throwing and catching while balancing.
To develop cooperation.

Equipment:

Balance boards (see "Improvising Equipment" in Chapter X).
Beanbags and playground balls.

Method:

This activity is best done by a small group while the rest of the class has
   another activity.
Free spacing, each child with a board.

> *"Let me see you balance on your board...*
> *Try not to wobble...*
>
> *Spread your arms wide to help you...*
> *Now see if you can rock your board from side to side without falling off..."*

Repeat, rocking forward and backwards, with beanbag on head, squat
   down, turn around slowly, toss beanbag in air and catch, bounce a ball
   beside board.

With Partner:

Children balance on boards, facing each other a few feet apart.
Toss beanbag or ball back and forth.
Bounce ball back and forth.

WANDS

Objectives:

To increase cardiovascular efficiency, agility, coordination, and flexibility.
To exercise muscles of the whole body.
To develop awareness of direction.
To introduce prepositions in an informal and concrete way.

Equipment:

Wands made from ½″ or ¾″ wooden dowelling about 1 yard long or broom handles.
Milk cartons (weighted with sand) or cones with flat tops.

Method:

(Note: Children must not be allowed to run around with wands, as they might stick them into other children.)
Maintain good spacing.
This activity is best done by a small group while the rest of the class has another activity.
Place wands on ground.
Use for prepositional challenges (see "Hoops" in this chapter).
Place across the top of milk cartons or cones.
Use as hurdles to leap, jump, hop over, crawl under, slither under like a snake, worm, or crocodile, on back, on tummy, on side.
Use mats if surface is rough.
Alternate, leap over, slither under.
Use in an obstacle relay.

PARACHUTE

Objectives:

To increase muscular strength, particularly in the upper body, arms, and hands.
To increase agility.
To stimulate the imagination.
To encourage cooperation.
To develop courage.

Equipment:

Parachute (often available from military surplus stores).
Beanbags.
Balls: Ping Pong,™ playground, whiffle, yarn.

Method:

(Note: Do not have parachute play on a windy day.)
Children must hold parachute tightly.

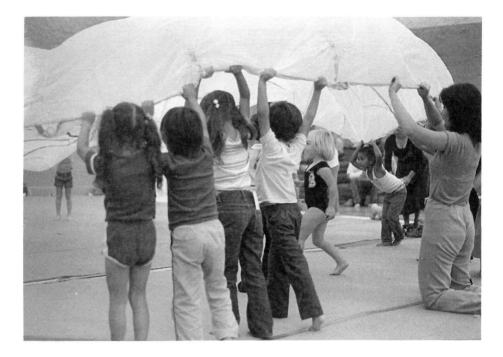

Figure 10. "Make a circus tent."

They must watch out for others when moving under it.
Spread parachute flat on ground.
Space children evenly around it.
Show them how to grip the parachute by the rolled edge.

> *"Grip like an eagle holding on to his perch . . .*
> *Now stand up and pull the parachute towards your tummy to make a big*
> *   flat pancake . . .*
> *Now we are going to make little waves by gently shaking the chute up and*
> *   down . . . "*

Repeat, making big waves with more vigorous shakes.
Throw several Ping-Pong or whiffle balls on top and make waves to send
    them through the middle hole or over the side.

> *"Let's make hailstones bounce up and down . . .*
> *Let's pop popcorn . . . "*

Designate at least three children to retrieve runaway balls.
Pretend two beanbags, or yarn balls, are rafts going through rapids.

> *"Try to help the rafts all the way around the chute . . . "*

Throw three jump ropes, or elastic ropes, on top of parachute.

> *"Pretend that these are wiggly worms.*
> *Shake the chute and send them down the middle hole . . . "*

Have children squat and hold chute.
Instruct them to stand and raise it above their heads, holding on tightly, to form a circus tent.
Lower to ground again.
Repeat, adding movements under the circus tent.

> *"All the girls run in, pretend you are a circus clown, and run out before the tent comes down . . .*
> *All the children wearing blue jeans run in and pretend you are a circus animal . . .*
> *Don't get caught in the tent!*
> *All the children wearing something red, run in and shelter from the rain . . .*
> *All the children wearing a barette run across under the tent before it comes down . . . "*

Put five beanbags in the center under the chute.

> *"All the boys pretend you are a dog . . .*
> *Run in, fetch a bone, and run home . . . "*

Instruct children how to make a mountain.
Grasp chute and raise it overhead.
Then quickly squat down and pull edge to ground.
Anchor it with hands and knees.
Repeat, adding movements for groups inside mountain, such as for under circus tent.
Do not leave children inside for more than a few seconds.
When children demonstrate they can keep a firm grip on the chute, add:

> *"Raise chute above head, take one step forward, turn to face outwards, change handgrip to inside and pull edge down to ground."*

All the children will now be inside.
Reverse all moves to get out again.
Instruct children how to make a mushroom.
Grasp chute, and raise it overhead.
Move to center to form a mushroom.
Move quickly back out to flatten it.

Instruct children how to make a merry-go-round.

Grasp chute and hold at waist level with two hands.

Slide in one direction, and on signal slide the other way.

Repeat, with half the class holding the chute while their partners stand behind them with hands on shoulders (horses and riders).

On signal "Up" or "Down," riders move to catch up with the next horse or wait for the next horse to come by.

Repeat, using other locomotor movements: Walk, run, jump, hop, skip, gallop, etc.

Use music to develop timing and rhythm sense.

LADDER

Objectives:

To develop agility, coordination, and balance.

To develop accuracy in throwing and catching while balancing.

To develop cooperation.

Equipment:

Ladder (wooden).

Carpet samples or mats.

Beanbags or balls.

Method:

This activity is best done by a small group while the rest of the class has another activity.

Have no more than six in a group.

Bare feet give the best grip on the ladder.

Maintain good spacing between children taking turns.

Place ladder flat on ground, with carpet samples or mats under the ends to avoid slipping.

> *"Today, let's try to walk along the ladder, putting our feet in the spaces. Try not to touch the rungs ..."*

Repeat, using jump, hop, walk backwards.

> *"This time let me see you walk slowly along the sides (rails) ...*
> *You will have to spread your legs wide (straddle walk) ..."*

Try not to fall off...
Now try to walk like a monkey using your hands and feet on the rungs... "

Place ends of ladder on rolled mats.

"Now we're going to take giant steps in the spaces, lift your knees high, and
try not to touch the rungs... "

Stand ladder on side; have two children hold ends to steady it.

"Let me see you crawl in and out of the spaces...
Climb over the ladder... you may use your hands to help you... "

With Partner:

Place ladder flat on ground.

Partners stand on ladder rails facing each other, hands joined.

They try to straddle walk along the rails, one moving backwards, and the other forward, then reverse.

One child straddle walks along the rails and tosses a beanbag or ball to his/her partner standing at the other end of the ladder.

Partners walk on rungs towards each other, meet in the middle, hold hands, try to balance on one leg, while changing the position of the other leg, then turn, and return to own end.

Repeat, using squat, holding hands, pass each other in the middle without falling off.

Chapter II

THROWING, CATCHING, AIMING, STRIKING ACTIVITIES, AND GAMES

Current research has shown that a young child needs to experience many different throwing, catching, aiming, and striking activities in order to establish patterns for these basic sports movements. It has also been observed that a soft, medium-sized ball leads to more success than a large playground ball which may make the child shy away. The color of the ball and the background may also have an influence on success. In one study, blue and yellow balls were caught more often than were white balls. Favorite-colored balls selected by the children were caught significantly more often.

The teacher should not hesitate to adapt the size, weight, or height of the equipment to the size of the children. Larger and lighter balls, plastic baseball bats, and lowered basketball rings will make for more chances of success in ball handling and skill improvement.

In this chapter the reader will find listings of the basic sports skills, and the progressions that a child should go through, in order to eventually take part in major sports activities with a *reasonable amount of skill.*

One of the most common occurrences in physical education programs is that the more skilled children tend to dominate their games, and the less skilled children receive little opportunity to improve their skills. A good teacher recognizes this and provides maximum opportunity for all children to throw, catch, aim, and strike balls, beanbags, rings, balloons, etc., as many times as possible during a lesson. No child ever improved in a skill by waiting for a turn to handle a ball. The aim is to have one ball per child for individual activities; one ball between two for pair activities.

PROGRESSIONS IN DEVELOPING SPORTS ABILITIES

Major Sports: Those games most often engaged in by adults on an organized basis or as recreational pursuits.

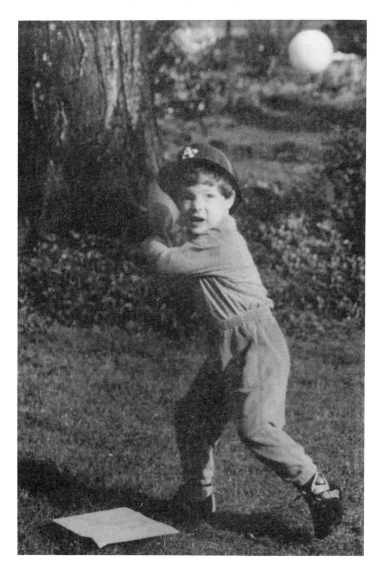

Figure 11. Use larger, lighter bats and balls.

Minor Games: Low organized games which use the skills of major sports, require very little equipment, involve more students, and have simple rules.

Relays: Small team activities, usually in lines, where students take turns; an element of speed is added.

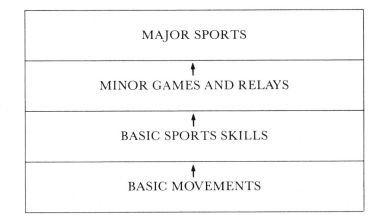

Basic Sports Skills:

Basketball	*Volleyball*	*Soccer*	*Softball*
Throw	Serve	Dribble	Catch
Catch	Dig	Pass	Throw
Dribble	Volley	Trap	Hit
Shoot	Spike	Shoot	Run Bases
Guard	Set-up	Tackle	Field
Strategy	Strategy	Strategy	Strategy
Rules	Rules	Rules	Rules
(Knowledge and Interpretation)			

Football	*Badminton*	*Tennis*	*Racquetball*
Throw	Serve	Forehand	Hit
Catch	Hit	Backhand	Rebound
Block	Clear	Serve	Serve
Kick	Strategy	Lob	Strategy
Strategy	Rules	Strategy	Rules
Rules		Rules	

Basic Movements: Walk, run, jump, hop, leap, bend, stretch, twist—adapted to a ball, bat, racquet, court, field, set of rules, time limit, teammate, and opponent.

BEANBAGS

Objectives:

To increase accuracy in throwing, catching, and aiming.
To manipulate the beanbag in many ways.
To involve the whole body in activity.

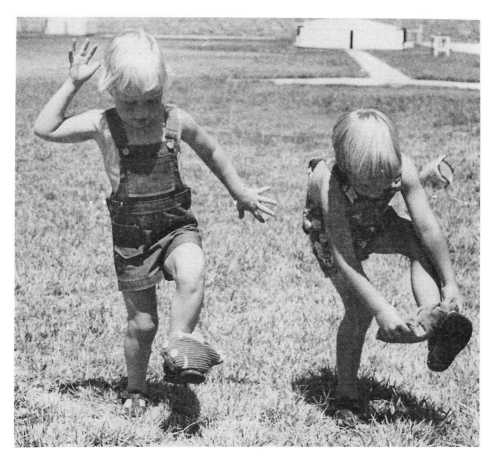

Figure 12. "Hop with your beanbag on your foot."

Equipment:

Beanbags (approximately 6″ × 6″) made from old jeans.
Skittles, milk cartons, cones.
Target box (see "Improvising Equipment" in Chapter X).

Method:

Have at least one beanbag for each child.
Free spacing, in designated area.

> *"Walk with your beanbag on your head ... under chin ... on the back of your hand ... "*

Repeat with chest, knee, armpit, elbow.

"Walk slowly ... fast ... high ... low ...
Hop with beanbag on your foot ...
Jump with beanbag between your feet ...
Walk with beanbag between your knees ...
Place it on your foot; kick it up and over head; kick it up and catch it ...
Place it behind knee; try to hop with it ...
Place beanbag between feet; jump it up to catch it ...
Crawl with beanbag on your back, forward ... backwards ...
Walk like a spider with beanbag on your tummy ...
Throw it up and catch with two hands ... hand to hand ... "

Repeat while children sit, kneel, stand, walk around.

"Throw as high as you can; try to catch it ... "
Throw high, clap hands before catching it ... "

Repeat with touch the ground, turn around, etc.

"Throw it as far as you can; run and fetch it ...
Place beanbag on the floor, pick it up with your toes, and hop ... "
(Children must be barefooted.)

"Bunny jump with beanbag between your feet ...
Lie on the floor with beanbag between your feet, try to lift it over your
*   head ... and put it on the floor behind your head ...*
*   bring it back again ...*
Place beanbag between your feet, forward roll and keep it there ... "

Repeat with backward roll.

"Place your beanbag on the floor, keep one hand on it, try to move around
*   it like a compass ...*
Throw your beanbag at the target on the wall ...
Throw your beanbag at the target ... "
(Use skittle, milk carton, cone.)

"Throw your beanbag into the target box ... "

With Partner:

"Throw and catch with your partner; use two hands, one hand ... "

Start sitting down, kneeling, standing up, moving around.

"Can you throw your beanbag with your toes ... knee ... elbow? ...
Exchange beanbags with your partner in different ways ... "

Lift it with foot to partner, toss it back over head, kick it back over head,
   toss it between legs.

In Threes:

Slide beanbag under bridge, made by child in push-up position.
Throw beanbag over the top of bridge.
Play "Piggy in the Middle," where child in center tries to intercept.

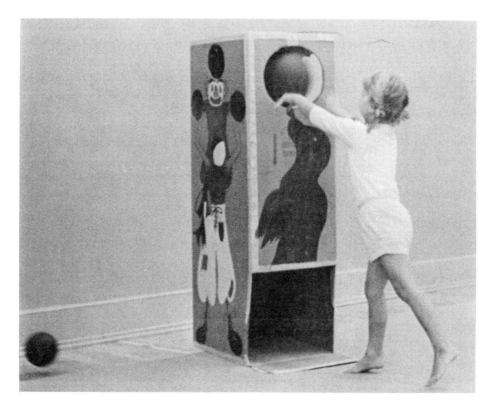

Figure 13. Target box: decorated carton.

TARGET BOX

Objectives:

To increase accuracy in throwing, kicking, rolling, and aiming.
To recognize geometrical shapes.
To practice addition and subtraction.

Equipment:

Large grocery cartons, decorated by the children

Cut circles, squares, triangles, rectangles in sides of cartons (see "Improvising Equipment" in Chapter X).

Method:

This is a good small-group activity.

Have children run and retrieve beanbags, etc., out of box.

Count how many went in and how many went out.

Toss beanbags or balls into circle, square, etc., underhand, overhand.

Move target box back as children have success.

Roll ball along ground into rectangle (soccer goal).

Kick ball into rectangle.

Place target box on a desk or table to raise the level.

Use like a basketball goal.

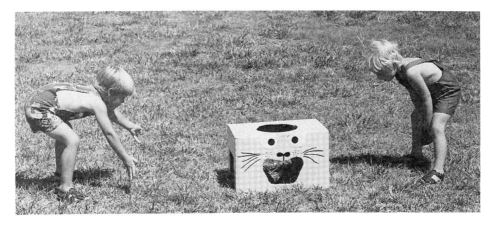

Figure 14. "Toss your beanbag into the target box."

CLOWN FACE

Objectives:

To increase accuracy in throwing and aiming.

Equipment:

Large cardboard clown face with cutout mouth attached to wall (see "Improvising Equipment" in Chapter X).

Method:

This is a good small-group activity.
Have children stand behind a line close to the target.
Move them back to other lines as they become more skilled.
Toss beanbag or balls to see if they can go through the mouth.
Have children run and retrieve beanbags, etc.
Count how many went in and how many missed.

WALL TARGET

Objectives:

To increase accuracy in throwing and aiming.

Equipment:

Large cardboard targets attached to wall or drawn on wall (see "Improvising Equipment" in Chapter X).

Method:

Same as for "Clown Face."
Have children add up their scores.

WALL BASKETS

Objectives:

To increase accuracy in throwing and aiming.

Equipment:

Use medium-sized grocery cartons with bottoms cut out or commercial basketball goals.
Attach to wall at different levels.

Method:

This is a good small-group activity.
Have children stand close to first low basket and try to shoot a basket with a beanbag or ball.
After two tries, successful or not, move to the next level basket.
Count how many baskets are made.

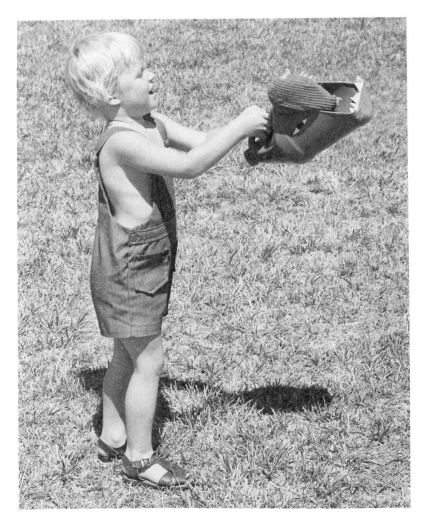

Figure 15. "Toss and catch your beanbag."

BLEACH BOTTLE CATCHERS

Objectives:

To increase accuracy in catching and stopping ground balls.
To simulate a catcher's mitt.

Equipment:

Make catchers out of bleach bottles and have children decorate them (see
  "Improvising Equipment" in Chapter X).
Use plastic balls, foam balls, yarn balls, old tennis balls, beanbags, etc.

Method:

Free spacing, with plenty of room between children to avoid collisions.

> *"Put your ball in your catcher...*
> *Can you toss it up in the air and catch it?...*
> *Use two hands, then one hand...*
> *Try to toss it higher...*
> *Can you walk while you toss and catch your ball?...*
> *Can you let your ball bounce once before you catch it?...*
> *Let me see you toss your ball across the playground...*
> *Run and get it and try again..."*

With Partner:

> *"Let me see you toss and catch the ball with your friend...*
> *Now stand further back and do it...*
> *Can you make your friend reach high for it?...*
> *Now low to the side...*
> *See if you can stop your friend's ball as it rolls along the ground...*
> *Scoop it up in your catcher...*
> *Can you toss your ball backwards over your head to your friend?...*
> *Now can you walk and toss and catch at the same time?...*
> *Try not to bump into anyone..."*

FRISBEE—COFFEE CAN LIDS

Objectives:

To increase accuracy in tossing, catching, aiming.

Equipment:

Use plastic coffee can lids of various sizes.
Have children decorate them.
Foam discs are available commercially.

Method:

Free spacing, with plenty of room between children to avoid collisions.
Have children toss lids freely into the air, run and retrieve them, and
toss again.
Stress keeping eyes open to avoid bumping into each other.
Toss lids into laundry baskets, hoops, etc.

With Partner:

Toss and catch with partner.
Increase distance between children.

In Groups:

Teacher tosses many lids into air.
Children retrieve as many as they can and count them.

BALLS

Objectives:

To increase accuracy in throwing, catching, and aiming.
To develop ball-handling skills for participation in ball games and
sports.

Equipment:

Large, medium, and small playground balls; soft balls made from yarn,
nylon stockings; fleece balls, plastic whiffle balls; old playground balls
stuffed with newspapers; tennis balls, foam balls.

Method:

Have at least one ball for each child.
Line balls up alongside designated area.
On signal, have children run to get ball, find their very own space, and
place ball between feet so it won't run away.
Have a stop signal (whistle, clap hands, "STOP") so that children know
to always put ball between feet when they hear it.

> *"Can you roll your ball along the ground and walk beside it? . . .
> Can you roll it sideways? . . ."*

Repeat with backwards and in a circle.

"Let's try to bounce and catch our balls...
Make a basket with your hands, open the basket, and let the ball fall...
Bounce your ball and catch it...again and again...
Throw your ball up in the air and catch it...throw...catch...throw...
*   catch...*
Throw your ball up in the air and try to turn around before it touches the
*   ground..."*

Repeat with try to touch the ground.

"Bounce your ball hard and do what it does until it stops moving...
Can you walk around and throw and catch your ball?...
Let me see you pat the ball with two hands..."

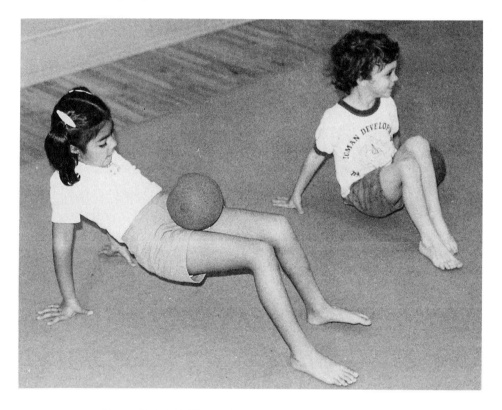

Figure 16. "Walk like a spider with the ball on your tummy."

Repeat with one hand, other hand, while walking, running, skipping, jumping, turning around, changing levels.

"Now can you bounce your ball while you say this rhyme?

> 'See how I can bounce my ball
> Never, never let it fall
> One and two and three and four
> Hold it tight and sit on the floor'

Now throw your ball in the air as you say this rhyme.

> 'See how I throw up my ball
> Never, never let it fall
> One and two and three and four
> Hold it tight and stand up tall'

Let me see you move your ball with little kicks with the side of your foot...
Run beside your ball... don't let it get away!...
Now can you do big kicks with the top of your foot, where your shoelaces
    are?...
Kick your ball and try to race it to the wall..."
"Can you bounce your ball with your elbow?... forehead... knee...
Let me see you walk like a spider with the ball on your tummy..."

Repeat with forward, backwards, sideways.

"Put your ball between your knees and jump forward... backwards...
Put it between your feet and jump up and down..."

Repeat, with forward, backwards, turning around.

"Can you bunny jump and toss the ball over your head?...
Lie on your back with your ball between your feet, toss the ball into the air
    and catch it with your hands...
Now let me see you make your ball do three different things..."

Have children demonstrate for each other.

With Partner:

Sitting on floor opposite partner with legs wide.
Roll ball back and forth, throw and catch.
Repeat, kneeling and standing, increase distance between partners.
Bounce ball to partner.
Throw ball between legs.
Roll ball to each other between legs.
Roll ball to be stopped by partner's feet, legs.
Have partner dodge rolled ball.
Throw ball so partner has to jump to catch it.

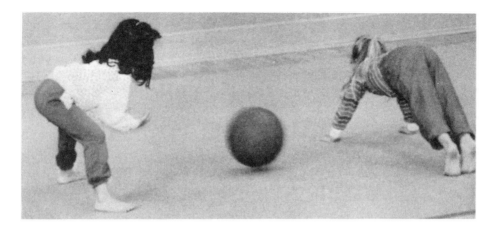

Figure 17. "Roll the ball under the bridge."

Throw ball over a suspended rope or through a hoop.

Bounce ball through partner's legs and run behind to retrieve it.

One child holds arms out to make a basket, partner runs up, makes basket, lets ball touch the ground before running back to place.

"Siamese Twins," partners put ball between heads (sides) and try to move forward without losing the ball.

In Threes:

"Piggy in the Middle"—one child in center tries to intercept ball.

"Under the Bridge"—roll ball under the bridge, made by child in push-up position; toss the ball over the bridge while child is in lowered position.

BALLOONS, BEACH BALLS, VOLLEYBALLS

Objectives:

To manipulate the balloon with hands or racquet.

To develop hand/eye coordination.

To increase awareness of the lightness of the balloon.

Equipment:

One balloon for each child and several spares for the inevitable bursting.

Goodminton racquets, rolled up newspapers, sticks.

Light, soft volleyballs, or beach balls can also be used.

Method:

> *"Let me see you pat your balloon with your hand ... now the other*
> *hand ...*
> *Try to keep it in the air ...*
> *Count how many pats you make ... "*

Repeat, with right hand, left hand, both, with fingers only.
Use racquets, sticks.

With Partner:

Have children pat the balloon back and forth.
Repeat, over a rope, through a suspended hoop.
Repeat, with beach balls, then light volleyballs.
Use racquets, sticks.

In Groups:

Have children pat the balloon around and across the circle.

PLASTIC BASEBALL BATS AND TEES

Objectives:

To develop hand/eye coordination.
To develop batting skills for minor games and major sports.

Equipment:

Small, lightweight plastic baseball bats; plastic bowling pins; batting tees
    or traffic cones; plastic whiffle balls; playground balls; "nerf" balls.

Method:

(Note: Good spacing must be maintained between children.)
Set out as many tees as possible along a line.
Have children place ball on top.
On the signal "Hit," they all hit their balls forward.
On the signal "Go," they all run forward to retrieve their balls.
The next children move up to the tees for a turn.
Progress to playing Tee Ball.

GOODMINTON

Objectives:

To develop hand/eye coordination.
To develop striking skills for racquet sports.

Equipment:

Goodminton racquets made from old pantyhose and wire coat hangers (see "Improvising Equipment" in Chapter X).
Balls made from pantyhose, crumpled up newspapers; whiffle balls, balloons, Ping-Pong balls.

Method:

Have children pat their balls in the air.
Count how many pats.
Bat the balls along the ground, run after them and bat again.
Suspend balls on strings from a horizontal rope.
Have children bat their balls forehand and backhand.

With Partner:

"How many times can you pat the ball back and forth with your partner?... (over a rope)

Try to keep your ball in the air..."

MINI-TENNIS

Objectives:

To develop hand/eye coordination.
To develop striking skills for racquet sports.

Equipment:

Plastic tennis type racquets with short handles.
Wooden bats, commercially produced or made from plywood (see "Improvising Equipment" in Chapter X).
Balls: foam, whiffle, yarn, Ping-Pong.

Method:

Have children pat their balls in the air.

Count how many pats.

Catch ball on the other side of racquet; pat ball up with that side.

Repeat, walking forward.

Suspend balls on strings from a horizontal rope.

Have children bat the balls forehand and backhand.

Bat the balls along the ground, run after them, and bat again.

Bat the balls against a wall.

Count how many pats before the ball touches the ground.

With Partner:

Have children pat the ball back and forth.

Count how many pats before the ball touches the ground.

Repeat over a low net or rope.

Count how many times the ball crosses the net.

RINGS

Objective:

To increase accuracy in tossing and rolling.

Equipment:

Deck tennis rings, rope rings, foam or plastic rings, garden hose rings, preserving jar rings, plywood board with cup hooks, rolled up magazines, relay batons, wooden dowel targets, hoops, plastic clothes baskets, inverted chairs.

Method:

> *"Let me see you toss the rings at the target...*
> *See how many you can get on the hooks..."*

In the basket, or hoop, or on the chair legs.

> *"Can you bowl your ring along the ground and run beside it?..."*

Repeat with race it to the wall, leap over it, run around it.

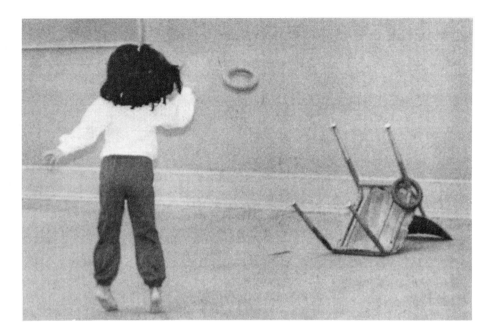

Figure 18. "Toss the ring on the chair leg."

With Partner:

Have one child hold rolled up magazine or relay baton vertically while
    other child tries to toss the ring on to it.
Increase distance from target.
Bowl rings back and forth.

In Threes:

Play "Piggy in the Middle."
Bowl ring between legs of child standing astride in the middle.
Have child in middle jump over bowled ring.

HANDSIE

Objective:

To increase manipulative skill and agility.

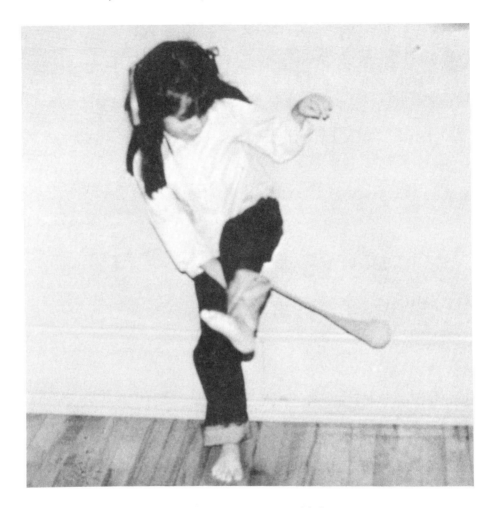

Figure 19. Playing "Handsie."

Equipment:

Tennis ball, in toe of knee-high hose or cutoff pantyhose leg (see "Improvising Equipment" in Chapter X).

Method:

Child stands against wall with hose in right hand.

Swings ball in hose, across body, to hit wall on left side of body, swings it back to hit wall on right side of body, at the same time raising left leg to a horizontal or higher position up wall; swings ball across body to hit wall below raised leg.

Repeat as many times as possible.
Repeat, with left hand, and raise right leg.

FOOTSIE

Objective:

To increase agility and coordination.

Equipment:

Commercially produced footsie rings and balls or plastic ring cut from base of bleach bottle and attached to old tennis ball with a length of string (see "Improvising Equipment" in Chapter X).

Method:

Have child place ring on right ankle.
Swing ball sideways and forward in a wide, counterclockwise circle, step on right foot, and leap over string with left foot.
Repeat, moving forward.

With Partner:

Partner stands ready to jump, leap, or hop over string as it circles.

In Threes:

Increase the length of the string.
Two children jump over the string as it circles.

JUGGLING

Objectives:

To develop hand/eye coordination.

Equipment:

Nylon scarves, plastic rings, juggling cubes, and balls.

Method:

Have children toss up and catch one scarf at a time, in right hand.
Repeat with left hand.
Now toss scarf in a high arch from right to left hand.

Repeat from left to right.

Have children alternately toss two scarves in the air and catch.

Now have children try to toss scarves high in an arc to pass in the air and be caught in the opposite hand.

Once children have had success with the scarves, repeat the above activities with rings, cubes, and balls.

SKITTLES

Objectives:

To develop hand/eye and foot/eye coordination.

To increase accuracy in aiming at a target.

Equipment:

Skittles, made from milk cartons, or bleach bottles half filled with sand.

Traffic cones or old bowling pins.

Balls: yarn, playground, whiffle.

Beanbags.

Method:

Set up a group of skittles close enough for the children to have immediate success.

Have children roll, toss, kick, balls at skittles.

Count how many went down and how many stayed up.

Increase the distance between children and skittles.

RELAYS

(Note: In a relay you are introducing the elements of speed and competition.)

This may have a deteriorating effect on a young child's performance.

Do not introduce relays too soon.

De-emphasize the competitive aspect to start with.

Keep team sizes small so children are not waiting in line for a turn (six is a good size).

Repeat the relay several times so children can have extra practice at skills.

Change leaders frequently to give all children a "moment of glory."

Have children squat (crouch) at the end of a relay so teachers can see who finished first.

Tunnel Ball Relay

Equipment:

Playground balls.

Method:

Children stand behind leader, with legs apart and bent forward.

On "go," leader rolls ball back between legs of children, who help it along if it stops.

Back child runs with ball to front of line to repeat the process.

The relay is ended when leader is back at the front of the line and all children are in a squat position.

Variations: Back child crawls through the tunnel of legs to the front.

Back child straddle-steps over children, who squat down as soon as ball passes under them.

Overhead Relay

Equipment:

Playground balls, yarn balls, beanbags.

Method:

Children stand behind leader with arms stretched overhead.

On "go," leader passes ball overhead to the next person in line.

Back child runs with ball to front of line to repeat the process.

The relay is ended when leader is back at the front of the line and all children are in a squat position.

Variations: Same as for "Tunnel Ball Relay."

Bob Ball Relay

Equipment:

Playground balls, yarn balls, beanbags.

Method:

Children stand in line, facing leader, who is one yard away from the second child.

On "go," leader tosses ball to second child, who tosses it back and squats down.

Leader repeats this with all children.

Last child receives the ball and runs to the front to take the leader's place.

Old leader quickly moves to stand at the front of the receiving line.

The relay is ended when all children have had a turn at the front and are squatting in their original positions.

Soccer Dribble Relay

Equipment:

Playground balls, skittles, cones.

Method:

Children stand in line behind leader, who has ball at his/her feet.

On "go," leader kicks ball with side of foot forward towards the skittle and around it, picks up ball, and runs back to hand it to the next child.

The relay is ended when all children have had a turn and are squatting in their original positions.

Variations: Dribble ball both ways.

Skip, hop, jump back to place.

Basketball dribble.

(For additional relay ideas, see Chapter III).

GAMES

(Note: The following simple games utilize the sports skills of throwing, catching, aiming, and striking balls, beanbags, etc.)

They have been selected for their simplicity and their involvement of as many children as possible.

The tag games and low organized games have been selected because they require the children to react quickly, to increase agility, and to incite as well as excite them.

The element of cooperation, as well as competition, should be emphasized.

If teams are necessary, they should be evenly matched. The teacher should select the teams, to avoid the less skilled child being embarrassed by being chosen last.

Every effort should be made by the teacher to see that all the children have some success or elation during each game's session.

Team uniforms are expensive and unnecessary. A simple band of colored material, worn diagonally across the upper body, will distinguish the teams (see "Improvising Equipment" in Chapter X).

Keep The Basket Full

Equipment:

Old tennis balls, Ping-Pong balls, beanbags, coffee can lids.
Plastic clothes basket or grocery carton.

Method:

Teacher and helper(s) stand behind basket of balls.
Children spread out in designated area.
On "go," teacher and helper toss the balls up in the air in all directions.
Children run to retrieve balls one at a time and bring them quickly back to the basket.
The aim of the game is for the teacher to keep the basket empty and for the children to keep it full.

All In Dodge Ball

Equipment:

Two playground balls.

Method:

One half of the class forms a circle.
The other half stands inside the circle.
On "go," the children forming the circle *roll* the balls into the circle and try to hit the other children's lower legs. The children in the center dodge about. If their feet are hit, they must go outside the circle and bounce up and down ten times.
When all children are out or at a signal from the teacher, the children change places.
(Note: Do not allow the game to go on too long, with only a few children left in the center.)

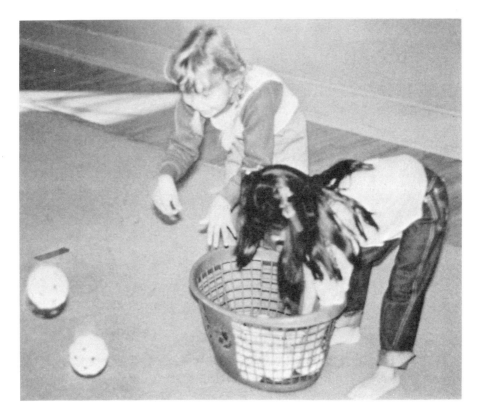

Figure 20. "Try to keep the basket full."

Knock The Tail Off

Equipment:

One or two playground balls.

Method:

Five children form a caterpillar in the center of a circle made by the
other children. They hold the waist of the child in front of them.

On "go," the children forming the circle *roll* the ball into the circle and
try to hit the lower legs of the last child forming the caterpillar, which
is dodging about to protect its tail.

If the last child is hit, (s)he leaves the circle and the second to last child
becomes the tail to be aimed at.

Repeat until all the children have been eliminated, then send in another
group.

Skittle Ball

Equipment:

Six playground balls, six milk cartons, or old bowling pins or traffic cones.

Method:

All the children form a circle around six skittles.
On "go," children with the balls try to knock down the skittles by rolling or kicking.
Children across the circle retrieve the balls and have a turn.

Jump The Beanbag

Equipment:

One beanbag tied securely onto a jump rope ten feet long.

Method:

Teacher or child in middle of a circle of children turns around and circles the rope and beanbag under the feet of the children, who must jump, leap, or hop over it as it comes towards them.
If a child is touched by the rope or beanbag, (s)he goes to the outside and bounces ten times before joining the class.
Change the center person frequently.

Rotten Eggs

Equipment:

One playground ball, tennis ball, or beanbag.

Method:

One child stands in the middle of a circle, throws the ball high in the air, and calls out the name of a child. The child who is called runs to retrieve the ball while the other children scatter. When the named child calls "stop," all the children must stand still. Then the named child looks to see which child is closest.
(S)he takes five large steps to get closer and tries to tag the other child with the ball. The tagged child becomes the one to start the game again.

Tee Ball

Equipment:

Batting tee, commercially produced or improvised (see "Improvising Equipment" in Chapter X).

Whiffle ball or playground ball.

Plastic bat or rolled up magazine.

Four beanbags for bases.

Method:

Children take turns hitting ball off tee and running to first base.

They wait on first base until next child hits and then run to second base.

This is repeated until they get home.

When this activity has been mastered, a fielding team and a batting team is formed.

Batter must get to first base before the ball is placed back on the tee.

Other runners must also get to their bases on time.

Teacher calls out "stop" and rules on whether runners are safe or not.

Chapter III

RACES, RELAYS AND CONTESTS

In races, relays, and contests, the element of competition is being introduced. This should not be overemphasized at the kindergarten and primary grade levels. Some young children thrive on competition; others experience their first taste of defeat and are turned off by the activity. Undue pressure to win can build up anxiety and result in a deterioration in performance. It is better to concentrate on the development of good basic skills than to introduce the element of competition too early. The emphasis should be on the children competing against themselves, to improve on their previous performances.

If competition against others is introduced, then careful consideration should be given to matching the competitors fairly in size, speed, strength, and agility, so that every child has a reasonable chance of success in each activity period.

If teams are to be used, the children should be grouped *by the teacher*, so that the strong will compensate for the weak, the fast for the slow, the agile for the clumsy. Pair activities could be equalized by having the big child propel the little child; the heavy child transport the light child.

The activities presented in this chapter can be used in the physical education period and then be incorporated into a mini track and field meet. In planning a meet, it is suggested that 75 percent of the activities be novelty and 25 percent traditional.

In novelty events, the elements of fun and luck are introduced so that the less skilled children have a chance to win. The traditional races can provide a challenge for the strong and fleet of foot.

All children should be included in at least one event in the meet, so that they have some involvement and can experience the elation of participation. It should be noted that it is easier to organize young children into races than into pairs or team relays.

MINI TRACK AND FIELD MEET PROGRAM

Novelty Events

Races:
- Beanbag on foot
  (behind knee, between knees)
- Piggies to Market
- Grocery Sack Race
- Shoebox Race
- Car Race
- Spider Ball
- Push the Peanut
- Ball Under Chin
- Skipping Rope
- Siamese Twins
- Ski Race

Novelty Relays:
- Potato
- Egg and Spoon
- Chain
- Caterpillar
- Ball Through Hoops
- Obstacle
- In and Out
- Oxford Boat Race
- City Gates
- Wheel

Traditional Events

Races:
- Run (25-, 50-, 75 yards)
- Skip (25 yards)

Relays:
- Shuttle (25-, 50 yards)

Jumps:
- Standing long jump
- Running long jump
- Team long jump
- High jump (scissors)
- Vertical jump

Hurdles:
- Low boxes, ropes (25-, 50 yards)

Throws:
- Beanbag
- Softball
- Football (mini)
- Playground ball
- Frisbee

NOVELTY RACES

Beanbag On Foot

Equipment:

One beanbag for each child.

Method:

On "go," children hop to finish line, trying to keep beanbag on foot.

Variations: Tuck beanbag behind bent knee.
Jump with beanbag between knees.

Piggies To Market

Equipment:

One playground ball and one rolled up magazine for each child.

Method:

On "go," children prod "piggie" (ball) with end of magazine towards finish line.

They cannot touch the ball with their hands.

Discourage hitting the ball.

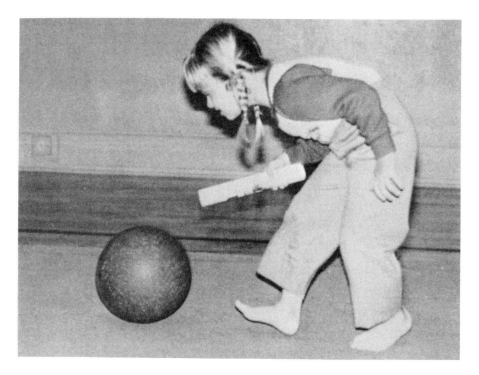

Figure 21. "Prod your piggie to market."

Grocery Sack Race

Equipment:

One grocery sack for each child.

Have plenty of spares to allow for tearing.

Method:

Children stand *behind* starting line with feet in sacks.
On "go," they jump to finish line.
They must finish with feet still inside sacks.

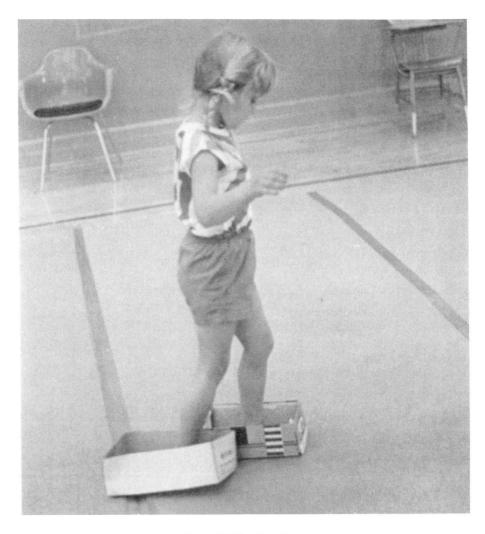

Figure 22. Shoebox Race.

Shoebox Race

Equipment:

Two shoeboxes for each child.

Method:

Children stand behind starting line with feet in shoeboxes.
On "go," they shuffle walk towards finish line.
They must finish with feet still in the boxes.
Variations: Use one box and have children hop.
Use one box balanced on head.
Use four boxes (two on feet and two on hands) and have children move
   on all fours.

Car Race

Equipment:

Large grocery carton with holes cut in top and bottom and decorated by
   children to look like a car.

Method:

Children stand inside their cartons and pull them up to waists.
Grasp sides of cartons.
On "go," children run to finish line, making car engine sounds.

Spider Ball

Equipment:

One playground ball for each child.

Method:

Children squat behind starting line with ball on tummy.
On "go," they spider walk on all fours towards finish line.
If balls fall off, they must stop and replace them.
They must finish with balls still on tummies.
Use short distances, e.g., 10 yards.

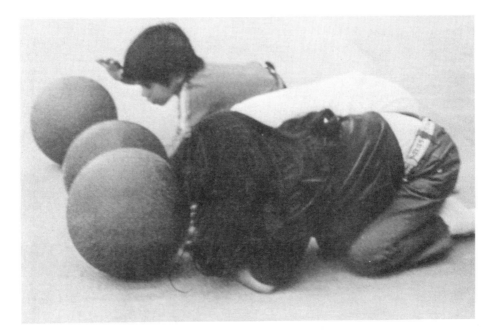

Figure 23. Push the Peanut Race.

Push The Peanut

Equipment:

One playground ball for each child.

Method:

Children kneel behind starting line with ball in front of them.
On "go," they crawl or move on all fours towards the finish line, "bunting"
   the ball with their forehead.
They cannot touch the ball with their hands.
Use short distances, e.g., 10 yards.

Kangaroo Race

Equipment:

One beanbag or playground ball, two plastic bowling pins, or rolled up
   magazines, for each child.

Method:

Children stand behind starting line, with ball or beanbag between knees (or thighs) and pins (or magazines) held up beside their ears to make large kangaroo ears.

On "go," they jump towards the finish line.

They must finish with ball between legs and ears in position.

Use short distances, e.g., 10 yards.

Ball Under Chin

Equipment:

One tennis ball, whiffle ball, or beanbag for each child.

Method:

Children stand behind starting line with ball under chin.

On "go," they walk fast, or run, towards finish line.

They must finish with ball under chin.

If it drops, they must stop and replace it.

Skipping Rope

Equipment:

One short rope for each child.

To gauge the right length, have children stand on the middle of the rope and see if it reaches from armpit to armpit.

Method:

On "go," children skip rope to finish line.

Use medium distances, e.g., 25 yards.

Siamese Twins

Equipment:

One playground ball for each pair.

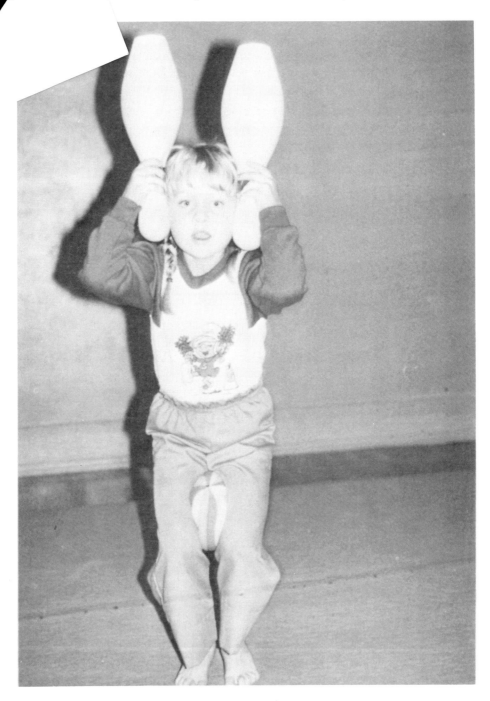

Figure 24. Kangaroo Race.

Method:

Partners stand back to back, side onto starting line, with ball between their upper backs and arms folded across their chests.

On "go," they slide sideways towards the finish line.

They must finish with ball in place.

If ball is dropped, they must stop to replace it.

Use short distances, e.g., 10 yards.

Ski Race

Equipment:

One grocery sack for each pair.

Method:

This is a good race to pair up a large child with a small child.

Small child stands on flattened grocery sack, facing large child, who has his/her back to the finish line.

On "go," large child grasps small child's hands and pulls him/her towards the finish line, being careful not to pull him/her off the grocery sack, which is being used like water skis.

NOVELTY RELAYS

Potato Relay

Equipment:

Five pebbles (or beanbags) for each team of six, placed one yard apart in front of starting line.

Method:

Teams sit in lines behind starting line.

On "go," the first team member runs to gather up the nearest "potato" and brings it back to the front of the team.

This is repeated until all "potatoes" are in front of the team.

Then the second team member takes the "potatoes" one at a time and places them back one yard apart.

This is repeated until all team members have had a turn, either gathering in the "potatoes" or spacing them out.

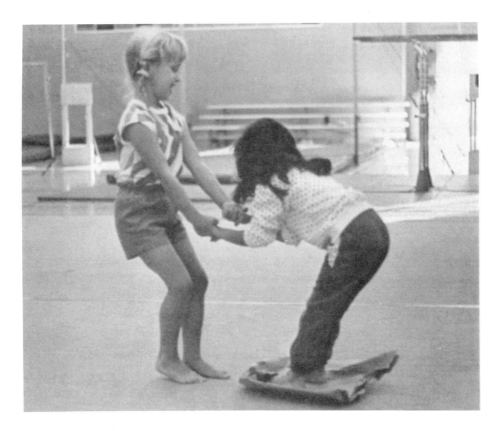

Figure 25. Ski Race.

Egg And Spoon Relay

Equipment:

One boiled egg (or pebble) and one plastic spoon for each team.

Method:

Half the team of six sits at one end of the relay area and the other half at
the opposite end.

On "go," the first team member carries the "egg" on the spoon to the
second team member, who in turn carries it back to the third team
member.

This is repeated until all team members have had a turn carrying the
"egg."

Chain Relay

Method:

Teams of six sit in lines behind the starting line.

On "go," the first team member runs to touch the ground (or beanbag) at the finishing line and runs back to reach out and grasp the right hand of the next team member. They run until the leader can touch the line again.

They then run sideways back to the team and the second team member reaches out to grasp the right hand of the next team member.

This is repeated until all team members have been gathered up into the "chain."

The winning team is the one whose last person crosses the finish line first with the "chain" intact.

Caterpillar Relay

Method:

Teams of six stand in lines behind the starting line with left hands on left shoulders.

On "go," they grasp the right knee of the person behind them, with their right hand, to form a "caterpillar."

"Caterpillar" hops on left feet towards the finish line, shouting "Hop! Hop!"

The winning team is the one whose tail (last person) crosses the finish line first.

Use short distances, e.g., 10 yards.

Ball Through Hoops Relay

Equipment:

One ball, three hoops for each team of six.

Method:

Three children stand evenly spaced between the starting and finishing lines, holding hoops up high and to the side of their heads.

Teams sit in lines behind starting line.

On "go," the first team member runs, carrying the ball, tosses it through each hoop, and runs back to give it to the next team member.

This is repeated until all children have had a turn and are back sitting in place.

Change hoop holders frequently.

Obstacle Relay

Equipment:

One playground ball, one short rope, one tumbling mat, one hoop for each team of six.

Method:

Place hoop 5 yards from starting line, make tumbling mat into a teepee or tunnel 5 yards from hoop, place short rope 5 yards from mat and ball 5 yards from rope.

Teams sit in lines behind starting line.

On "go," the first team member runs to hoop, passes it over his/her body, replaces it on the ground, runs to crawl under mat, runs to short rope and jumps three times, runs to ball, bounces it three times and replaces it on the ground, and runs back to tag the second team member.

This is repeated until all team members are back sitting in place.

In And Out Relay

Equipment:

One beanbag or ball for each team of six.

Method:

Teams stand in line, one yard apart, behind leader.

On "go," beanbag is passed down the line to the last team member, who runs forward, in and out of the team members, to become the leader.

All children move back one space.

This is repeated until all team members have come to the front and are back in place.

Oxford Boat Race

Method:

Teams squat in line with hands on the waist of the person in front; team leader stands facing the second team member and grasps his/her hands. This forms a "boat and crew."

On "go," team jumps forward in squat position and, in unison, shouting "Long! Short! Long! Short!", as they take a large jump followed by a jump on the spot.

The winning team is the one whose last crew member crosses the finish line first with the boat still intact.

Use short distances, e.g., 5 yards.

City Gates Relay

Method:

Four teams of six stand behind an "arch" made by two children at the corners of a square area.

On "go," the teams run through their own arches and forward to run through the other teams' arches at the corners of the square and finish in squat in their starting position.

Wheel Relay

Equipment:

One ball or beanbag for each of four teams.

Method:

Teams of six form the spokes of a wheel and stand side by side, with the leader at the center holding the ball.

On "go," the ball is passed along the team to the outside team member, who runs forward around the outside of all the teams (counterclockwise), in behind his/her own team to become the team leader, and passes the ball along the team again to the outside person.

Team members take one step outwards each time they handle the ball.

This is repeated until all children have had a turn at running with the ball.

TRADITIONAL EVENTS

RACES

Have starting and finish lines clearly defined, preferably with lines on the ground.

If using a finish tape, use pure-wool yarn that will break easily if the children holding it do not release it when the first child runs through.

Do not use tape, ropes, or any material that might cut into the first child to finish.

Never tie any of the above materials to posts.

Have efficient adult or senior level students to line up children and to see that they start from *behind* the starting line.

Begin early to disqualify those children who edge over the starting line.

Have efficient judges to see that the children who do finish first are indeed declared the winners.

It is a good idea to have children wear colored cloth bands diagonally across their bodies so that they can be distinguished by the judges.

RELAYS

The "shuttle" relay is the most appropriate relay for young children.

The distance can be varied.

Half the team lines up at one end of the relay area and the other half at the opposite end.

It is a good idea, with young children, to have them carry a beanbag or a rolled up magazine to exchange with the next runner.

Care must be taken to see that children do not edge over the starting line.

Judging is made easier by having the teams squat or sit to finish.

JUMPS

Standing Long Jump

Method:

Children stand at edge of pit, or behind a line, on the grass or tumbling mat.

They give two preliminary arm swings and body dips and then jump forward as far as they can.

The jump is measured from the starting line to their heel marks or whatever body mark is closest to the starting line.

Running Long Jump

Method:

It is best to use a pit filled with sand or sawdust for this event.

For young children, have them run up to the edge of the pit and take off (leap).

The jump is measured the same as for the standing long jump.

Team Long Jump

Method:

Teams of six line up behind the starting line.

Team leader does a standing long jump from the starting line.

The next team member stands where (s)he landed and jumps forward.

This is repeated until all children have had a turn.

The total distance jumped by the team is measured.

This is a good activity for teams to be composed of strong and weak jumpers.

High Jump (Scissors)

Method:

A grassy area or pit is needed for this event.

Have two children loosely hold a length of pure-wool yarn across pegs on two upright stands.

Instruct them to release the yarn if the jumper gets caught in it.

Instruct jumpers to approach the "crossbar" from the side and to scissors leap sideways over the yarn.

Move the pegs up to challenge the jumpers.

When teaching the scissors jump, a short rope held loosely by two children in a kneeling position can be used.

Vertical Jump

(See Chapter VI for "Nosey Parker Peek.")

HURDLES

Use low grocery cartons or short ropes held loosely by two children
 kneeling.
Space them evenly between the start and finish lines.
Encourage children to leap over the boxes but to keep the body low.

THROWS

Have a clearly defined starting line which the children cannot step over.
Mark where the beanbag or ball lands with tongue depressors and write
 the childrens' names on them.
Allow the children three turns to try to improve on their performances.
Have efficient field judges to monitor the throws.

CONTESTS

The contests included in this section are activities that challenge the
individual child, partners, or teams in a fun way.

Teepees

Partners of equal size and weight sit back to back, with elbows linked and
 knees bent to chests.
They push against each other's backs to stand up and form a "teepee"
 without moving feet or unlinking arms.
They then try to sit down slowly.
This is repeated several times.

Jumping Circuit

One child sits on the ground with legs astride and arms held sideways at
 shoulder height or lower.
The other child leaps across the legs and over the arms in a jumping
 circuit.
Partners change places.

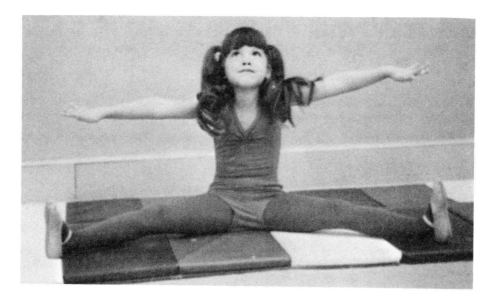

Figure 26. One child provides a jumping circuit.

Bridges

One child forms a bridge by taking a push-up position.
While the bridge is up, the other child crawls under it.
While it is down flat on the ground, the other child leaps or jumps over
  it.
Partners change position.

Dog And Bone

Partners stand opposite each other, behind lines, about 10 yards apart.
A beanbag is placed in the center of the area.
On "go," the children run to the beanbag and try to pick it up and take it
  back over their starting line without being tagged by their partner.

Lost Your Shadow

Partners stand one behind the other.
On "go," the child in front tries to dodge away from the child behind and
  not let him/her on the "shadow."

When the whistle blows, the "shadows" try to reach forward and touch
their partners.

Center Ball Exchange

Partners stand opposite each other and behind lines.
All the children behind one line hold a ball or beanbag.
On "go," the children run to the center and exchange balls with their
partners, who carry them back over the starting lines.

Beat Your Partner

Children stand in threes, holding hands, with the middle child standing
on a center line.
On "go," the two outside children run to touch the sidelines and back to
hold hands with the middle child.
The child who is last back changes places with the middle child.

RACING AND CHASING GAMES

Tails

Equipment:

Strips of material, one for each child.
Folded team bands may be used.

Method:

Children tuck "tails" into the back waistband of their shorts so that at
least 12 inches of tail is visible.

Shadows

Method:

(Note: A sunny day is necessary to play this game.)
Two children are designated as catchers.
On "go," other children scatter in area and catchers try to step on their
shadows.

Count how many shadows are stepped on.
Change catchers quickly.

What's The Time Mr. Wolf?

Method:

One child is designated as "Mr. Wolf."
Children walk across the playground behind him/her, calling out, "What's the time Mr. Wolf?"
Mr. Wolf calls out times and children clap that number.
When Mr. Wolf calls "Dinner time," (s)he turns and runs after children, who try to cross their home line before (s)he catches them.

Dry Feet, Wet Feet

Equipment:

A "stream" drawn on the playground, with wide and narrow parts (see "Playground Markings" in Chapter X).

Method:

Children form groups of six and play "Follow the Leader" by running and leaping across the stream wherever the leader leaps—sometimes in the narrow parts and sometimes in the wide parts. They try not to get their feet wet.
Change the leaders frequently.

Daisy Chains

Method:

All the children, except two, link elbows with a partner.
Of the two who are free, one is designated the catcher and the other the runner.
On "go," the catcher chases the runner, who can be saved by hooking elbows with either one of a couple. The partner of the child who is hooked on to then becomes the runner and must quickly run away to avoid the catcher. If a catcher tags a runner, the latter child becomes the catcher.
For large classes, there should be more catchers and runners.

Mr. Frost and Mrs. Thaw

Equipment:

A few white and red strips of material.

Method:

Two children are designated "Mr. Frost" and carry a white strip.

One child is designated "Mrs. Thaw" and carries a red strip.

On "go," other children scatter in designated area, trying not to be tagged by Mr. Frost.

If tagged, they must freeze on the spot.

They can only be unfrozen if tagged by Mrs. Thaw, then they are free to run again.

Change Mr. Frost and Mrs. Thaw frequently.

Cat and Mouse

Method:

One child is designated as "cat" and one child as "mouse."

The other children join hands to form a circle.

On "go," the cat chases the mouse in and out of the circle of children, who raise their arms to let the mouse through and lower them to hold the cat back.

If the mouse is tagged, a new pair is chosen.

Fox and Geese

Method:

In groups of six, one child is designated as the "fox."

The other children are geese and stand behind "Mother Goose" with arms around the waist of the child in front.

On "go," the fox tries to tag the last goose, while Mother Goose holds her arms out wide, and the line dodges back and forth to protect the last goose from the fox.

Circle Chase

Children stand in a circle.

Teacher gives them numbers, e.g., 1, 2, 3.

When teacher calls out a number, all the children with that number run
counterclockwise around the outside of the circle and try to tag the
runner in front of them without being tagged by the runner behind.

They are "safe" when back in their places.

Merry-Go-Round

Partners form a double circle.

Inside children join hands to form a merry-go-round.

Outside children place their hands on the shoulders of their partners.

On "go," the whole class slides, in unison, counterclockwise.

On "up," the outside children try to move up (counterclockwise) to put
their hands on the shoulders of the next child.

On "down," the outside children move down (clockwise) to the next
child's shoulders.

Shipwreck

Method:

Teacher explains the following commands and actions to the class.

When they are called out, children respond.

The last child to respond to each command must go to the side until the
game ends.

COMMAND	ACTION
Bow	Run to front of room
Stern	Run to back of room
Port	Run to left side of room
Starboard	Run to right side of room
Climb the rigging	Do action of climbing the rigging
Hit the deck	Lie face down on floor
Scrub the deck	On one knee, scrub the floor
Captain's coming	Stand to attention and salute

Streets and Lanes

Method:

Children stand in lines of six, facing *front,* with arms stretched sideways
to touch the next child.

Two children play chase up and down the "streets" made by the class.
They cannot go underneath the arms.

When teacher calls out "lanes," the class turns to face the *side* of the play area and the children playing chase must change direction and run up and down the "lanes."

Teacher alternates the commands "streets" and "lanes" frequently.

More children can play chase at the same time as the game becomes more familiar.

Chapter IV

BEGINNING TUMBLING AND GYMNASTICS

The natural movements of young children involve rolling over, crawling, creeping, stretching, wiggling, reaching and balancing. These are basic tumbling and gymnastics activities. Very young children love to be upended and rolled about. They are very flexible, as shown when they bite their toes. If this flexibility can be maintained, they shall have a considerable advantage in gymnastics in kindergarten and the primary grades.

Perhaps the weakest area in young children's bodies is the upper body and shoulder area. They need to be given activities in which they support their body weight in various positions, such as swinging from a rope or horizontal bar or doing bunny jumps.

Many of the activities in Chapter I are valuable for strengthening and conditioning the body for tumbling and gymnastics. This chapter presents simple, sequential activities, some without equipment, and some with equipment that can be improvised (see "Improvising Equipment" in Chapter X).

The most important factor in introducing tumbling and gymnastics is to anticipate danger to children and to avoid injuries and accidents. During a gymnastics lesson, the teacher should be at the station where an accident is most likely to occur and should always be in a position to observe the whole class and to intervene when necessary.

All activities should be done slowly at first. The teacher or helper should ease children through the movement. Constant verbal cues and encouragement is important.

Children should know the signal to "STOP!" (whistle or voice) and to react at once. They should be taught to lift, carry, and put down equipment carefully so that it is not damaged. In the process, they shall learn sound mechanics of movement. Children should not be allowed to play on equipment, nor should damaged equipment be used. Damaged equipment should be moved to an inaccessible place until repaired. All equipment should be in a safe condition, with no sharp or jagged edges or nails protruding. It should be locked away when not in use.

Spacing of equipment and children is necessary to avoid collisions. This necessitates clear traffic lanes between equipment when in use.

Mats should be placed where children might land. Where floor surfaces are suitable, children could work in bare feet. Socks are too slippery. Ballet slippers or light gym shoes are an improvement on outdoor footwear.

Method:

There are two main methods of teaching gymnastics: direct (traditional) and movement education.

Direct (traditional): The teacher presents traditional tumbling and gymnastics activities in a sequence from simple to complex. Each child performs the same movements.

Movement Education: The teacher presents a theme or idea for the children to interpret in movement. Each child may respond with a different movement. Chapter I leans heavily towards the movement education approach to physical education. In this chapter, emphasis moves towards the direct approach on the premise that users of this text will have had little, if any, exposure to movement education methodology involving gymnastics equipment. However, children should be encouraged early to combine movements into original sequences and to apply artistry.

It is important that children should not have to wait in line for a turn on the mat. Have no more than six children to a group mat. Give them an activity to do to get back in line.

Examples: Hop, jump, skip, spider walk, bunny jump, monkey walk, inch worm. If only one or two mats are available, have two groups at the mats and the rest of the class using hoops, beanbags, jump ropes, etc., in an adjacent area (see "Methodology" in Chapter IX).

GYMNASTICS FUNDAMENTALS

Climbing, hanging, rolling, curling, stretching, crawling, twisting, swinging, pushing, pulling, supporting, balancing.

All of the above movements are incorporated into the activities described below. Teachers should often refer to the above list to see that their children are indeed experiencing these movements. It is a good idea to check off weekly those movements that have been incorporated into the previous week's activities.

BEGINNING ROLLS

Objectives:

To develop tumbling ability and agility.
To accustom the children to being in inverted positions.
To exercise the whole body.

Equipment:

Individual tumbling mats or large group mats.

Method:

The following challenges represent a progression from simple to more difficult rolls.
As the children master a roll, they progress to the next challenge.
This may take minutes, days, or weeks, depending on the abilities of the children.

Hot Dog Roll

"Can you roll sideways like a foot-long hot dog?..."
(Child stretches whole body and rolls sideways.)

Watermelon Roll

"Can you roll sideways like a watermelon?..."
(Child bends knees to chest, hugs them, puts chin on chest and rolls sideways.)

Combination Rolls

"Can you roll sideways like a hot dog, and then like a watermelon, and then like a hot dog all the way along the mat?..."

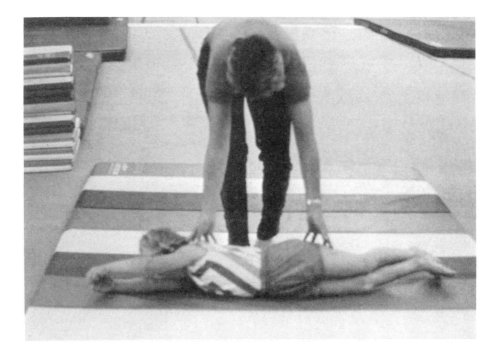

Figure 27. "Roll sideways like a hot dog."

Egg Roll

"Sit on the mat and hug your legs . . . now roll sideways, backwards and sideways like an egg . . . "

Shoulder Roll

"Squat facing the mat, put one hand on the mat . . .
try to roll over on your shoulder . . . "
(This is halfway between a watermelon roll and a forward roll.)

Forward Roll

To get the children into a good tuck position, use the following progressions:

"Squat like a bunny at the edge of the mat. With your knees wide apart, put your hands on the mat between your legs, tuck your head way under until you can see my hand behind you . . . "

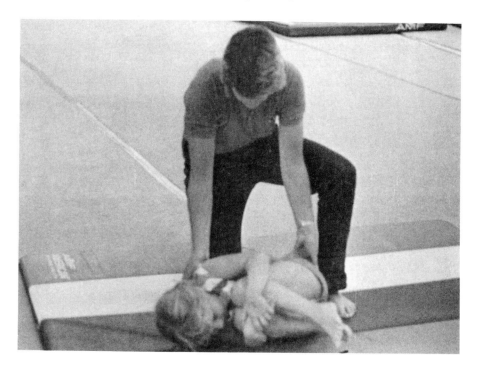

Figure 28. "Roll sideways like a watermelon."

Teacher places his/her left hand firmly on back of child's head and neck
   to maintain the tuck position and holds right hand behind child's seat
   where child can easily see it.
Teacher then raises right hand higher behind child.

   "Can you still see my hand? . . . "

Now the child has to really tuck his/her head away under and raise
   his/her seat up to still see the hand.
At this stage, gravity takes over and child goes into a forward roll.
   Teacher can assist by supporting child with left hand still at back of
   head and neck area and with right hand under seat.

Forward Roll Variations:

With feet together.
With beanbag between feet.
With legs wide.
From standing position to standing again.

Wheelbarrow walk with partner into forward roll.
Combine with backward roll.

Combination Rolls:

Combine rolls into a sequence along the mat and begin to include leaps, jumps and balances.

Examples: Hot dog, watermelon, egg, forward roll.

Hot dog, egg, forward roll, jump high in the air, balance on one foot for five counts.

Backward Roll

To get the children to attain a good curled-up position, use the following progressions.

Rocking Chair:

Child squats on mat, chin on chest, hugs legs, rocks backwards and forward.

Rock and Roll:

Child squats on mat, chin on chest, hands up like a traffic cop, rolls back until hands push on mat, returns to squat.

When a good curled-up position is maintained, child is encouraged to push hard on hands when they touch the mat and to roll over. Teacher helps by pulling *up* on child's hips to make room for the head.

Backward Roll Variations:

Wide astride sit to standing wide astride.
Wide astride stand to same position.
Push up to pike position at end of roll.

Combination Rolls:

Combine into a sequence using previously learned rolls, jumps, leaps and balances.

Headstand

To get the children to attain a good base of support, draw a head and hands on the mat to form a triangle. Make sure the hairline is on the

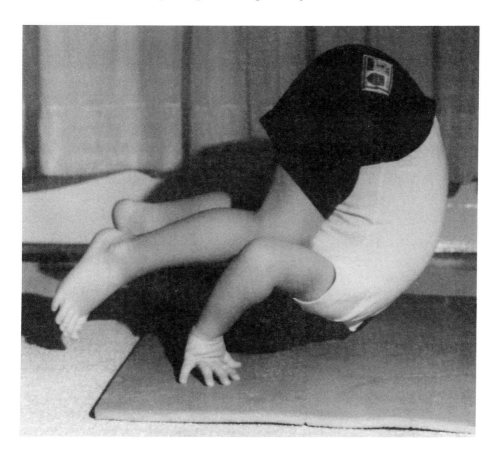

Figure 29. Gravity takes over and child goes into a forward roll.

mat, not the top of the head. This keeps the chin off the chest and prevents rolling over.

> *"Squat like a bunny at the edge of the mat. Put your forehead in the circle and your hands on the mat. Try to balance on your head and hands. Keep your knees bent close to your body..."*

Teacher stands on the mat, facing the child, and supports the hips.

> *"When you can balance, slowly straighten your legs...*
> *Now come down the way you went up..."*

Headstand Variations:

Tripod balance with knees on elbows.
Spread legs apart.

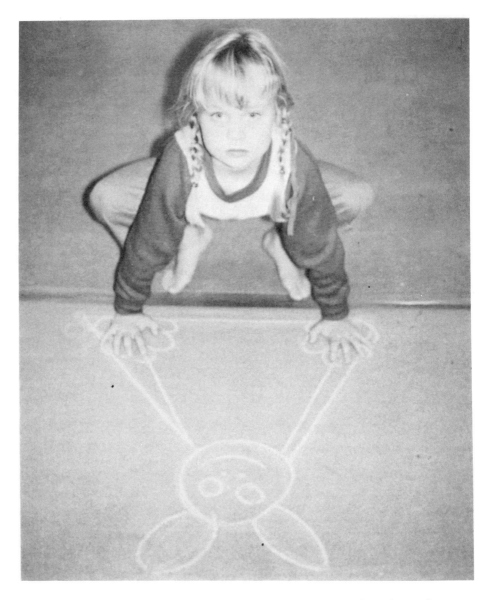

Figure 30. "Put your forehead in the circle and your hands on the mat."

Cross legs like a tailor.
Bicycle legs.
Tuck head under and forward roll.

Combinations:

Combine into a sequence using previously learned rolls, jumps, leaps, and balances.

Handstand

To develop upper-body strength, the children should use the following progressions:

Bunny Jump (Crouch Jump):

> *"Squat like a bunny at the edge of the mat, hands up by ears, and feet together. Press your hands on the mat and kick your feet up together to try to touch your seat...*
> *Keep your arms straight and look forward..."*

These bunny jumps may also be performed moving forward, with "front paws" reaching forward, and "back paws" following to catch up with "front paws."

No handstands should be attempted until the child demonstrates a strong bunny jump.

Donkey Kick:

> *"Squat at the edge with one leg bent and the other leg stretched behind you...*
> *Press your hands on the mat, look forward, and kick your legs up in the air like a donkey as many times as you can before you come down...*
> *Count how many kicks..."*

(Child kicks legs alternately.)

Mule Kick:

> *"Squat at the edge of the mat...*
> *Press your hands on the mat, look forward, keep your feet together, and kick them back and upwards like a frisky mule..."*

(Child kicks with feet together.)

Handstand in Fours:

One child takes donkey kick position between two children and in front of teacher. The extended back leg is kicked up strongly to attain a full handstand position. Child goes down the way (s)he came up.

Teacher supports hips and then extended legs.

Children kneel on one knee at side of performer and support under the shoulder with one hand and under the hips with the other.

Handstand in Twos:

When child has a strong position in previous progression, only teacher or one child supports hips and then legs.

Handstand Variations:

Balance against wall, change leg positions.
Free handstand without support.
Handstand balance, tuck head, forward roll.

Combinations:

Combine into a sequence using previously learned rolls, jumps, leaps and balances.

Cartwheel

The cartwheel is a handstand performed sideways, so it should be taught after the handstand is attained using the following progressions.
Bunny jump over a line or low rope.
Bunny jump as above but separate the legs.
The hands still press the floor together.
Straighten the legs during the movement and try to kick the ceiling.
The hands should go "pat" and the feet should go "pat, pat" as they land separately.
Start from standing position and keep the whole body extended during the cartwheel.

Combinations:

Combine into a sequence using previously learned rolls, jumps, leaps, and balances.

BEGINNING FLOOR EXERCISE

After the children have mastered a series of tumbling activities, the next step is to combine them into sequences. Then, simple beginning floor exercise routines can be developed, linking up tumbling moves with locomotor movements (walk, run, skip), and including leaps, jumps, ballet steps, held positions (arabesques, knee scales, attitudes, lunges, splits). As the children learn more difficult tumbling moves, they replace the simple ones in their routines.

A floor exercise area is not essential. Routines may be performed, back and forth, on a long mat area. Good form and artistic presentation is to be encouraged.

Floor Exercise Routines

1. Hot dog, watermelon, forward roll, backward roll, balance in arabesque, two skips forward, cartwheel, sideways splits.
2. Headstand, forward roll, jump high in the air, run forward, cartwheel, lunge sideways, backward roll to wide astride, forward roll to wide astride, jump feet together, attitude.

LOW BALANCE BEAM[1]

Low balance beams may be purchased or constructed (see "Improvising Equipment" in Chapter X).

The surface must be smooth and sliver free.

Barefeet should be encouraged for good traction.

Socks and street shoes are dangerous.

Do not allow running on the balance beam.

Have children hold teacher's hand or a friend's shoulder to begin with.

Encourage them to use their arms wide to aid balance.

Have them step down or jump off beam with control, even though it is low.

Do not have children in long lines waiting for a turn.

Let them progress at their own rate.

If no beam is available, most of the following activities can be performed along a line on the floor or the playground.

> *"Let me see you walk along the beam and step off...*
> *Now walk along the beam and jump off...*
> *Can you walk on your tiptoes and jump off?...*
> *Now are you ready to walk along on your own?...*
> *Stretch your arms wide to balance..."*

Place teddy bear at center of beam.

---

[1]Reprinted from *Instructor,* November 1973. Copyright© 1973 by the Instructor Publications, Inc. Reprinted by permission of Scholastic, Inc.

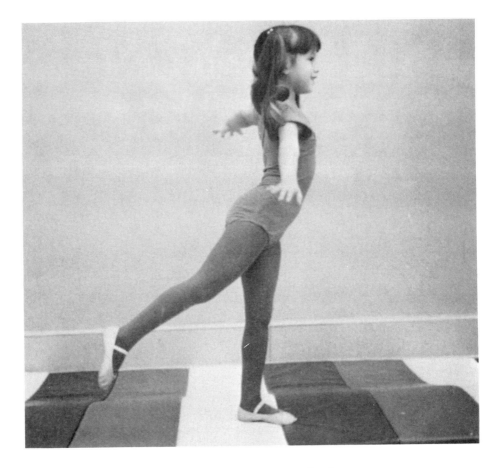

Figure 31. "Balance on one foot."

"Let me see you pick up Teddy and carry him to the end of the beam . . .
Now see if you can walk to the middle and balance on one foot . . . "

Repeat, using sit in the middle, lie down, sit up, stand up, walk to the end and jump off.

"This time let me see you walk sideways . . .
Now can you walk sideways on your own? . . .
Hold your tummy in and try not to wobble . . .
Can you walk backwards very slowly? . . .
Can you walk low? . . .
Can you walk like a monkey on all fours? . . .

Can you waddle like a duck?...
See if you can hop along on one foot...
Let me see you jump...
Let me see you take little skips..."

With Partner:

Teacher, or child, holds hoop *horizontally* at middle of beam at about knee height.

> *"Let me see you step into and out of the hoop...*
> *Now step into the hoop and crawl under it..."*

Teacher, or child, holds hoop or rope vertically at middle of beam.

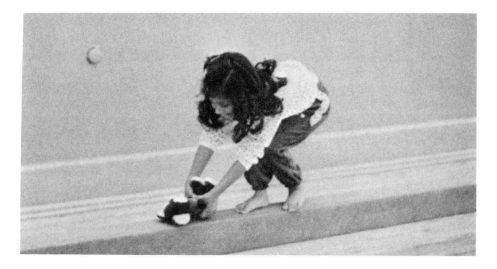

Figure 32. "Pick up the teddy and walk to the end."

> *"Can you creep through the hoop without touching it?..."*

Teacher, or child, stands at far end of beam with a beanbag or playground ball.

> *"As you walk along the beam, let me see you throw and catch the beanbag*
> *without falling off..."*
> *"Can you bounce your ball to the side of the beam as you walk along?...*
> *Let me see you throw your ball up in the air as you walk along..."*
> *"Can you slowly wheelbarrow your friend along the beam?..."*

Teacher asks child to put hands on the end of the beam, supports him/her *under thighs,* and asks him/her to walk along the beam on alternate hands while (s)he straddles the beam. Later, children can be matched for size and can wheelbarrow each other *very slowly.* At the end of the beam, the child who is the wheelbarrow walks on his/her hands off the beam on to a mat. Later they can tuck their heads under and forward roll, with friends still supporting.

> *"Put your hands on the beam...*
> *Show me how you can bunny jump over the beam...*
> *Keep your head up...*
> *Can you bunny jump all the way along the beam?... "*

HORIZONTAL BAR

Many playgrounds have low horizontal bars. These can be used by one group during a physical education lesson.

The teacher should be stationed there.

There must be a soft sandy surface underneath or a mat underneath the bars.

Have children grasp bar overhand and take their body weight.

Teacher places his/her hands over child's hands to maintain grip.

> *"Let me see you swing gently back and forth...*
> *Now can you swing with a very straight body and finish by hanging very still?...*
> *Can you swing along under the bar like a monkey?*
> (Child holds bar at end and kicks up legs to grip bar with them.)

> *"Can you perch like a bird on the bar?*
> (Child grasps the bar in overgrip, jumps to place upper thighs across bar, and tries to keep body upright and arched.)

> *"Now can you curl yourself around the bar and stand on the mat?... "*
> (Child bends at hips to encircle the bar, holding on tightly.)

The following moves are only to be attempted after the children have shown strength and confidence in the simple moves.

> *"Today we shall learn to 'Skin the Cat'... "*
> (Child grasps the bar in overgrip, brings legs bent up between hands, and rolls backwards to stand on mat and to release hands.)

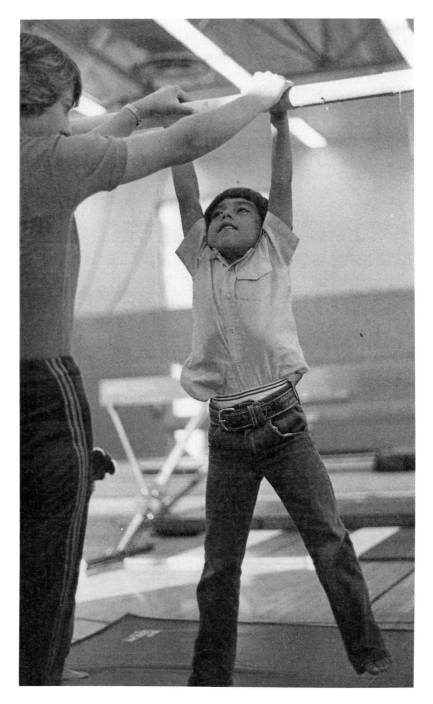

Figure 33. Teacher places hands over child's hands to maintain grip.

"Let me see you hang under the bar by your knees . . . "
(Teacher places hands across lower legs while child hangs or gently
    swings.
Child can regrasp bar and "Skin the Cat" or can place hands on mat,
    arms straight, and dismount through a handstand position.)

LOW VAULTING BOX

Small children can begin vaulting using the top layer of a vaulting box
or a constructed single- or double-layer box with a padded top (see
"Improvising Equipment" in Chapter X).

"See if you can bunny jump onto, along and off the box . . . "
(Child stands at end of box, places hands on, and bunny jumps to
    squat on the box, bunny jumps along and off to side.)

"This time try to bunny jump on and off the box . . . "
(Child stands to side of box and bunny jumps on to box and off to
    the other side.)

"Now you are ready to bunny jump over the box . . . "
(Child stands off to side of box and approaches it on the diagonal
    with a few steps, gives preparatory jump to bring feet together,
    places hands on the box, and bunny jumps over without feet
    touching it.)

"Let us now try a 'Hip Hump' . . . "
(Child stands back from side of box, steps forward, puts hands on
    box, and springs to land on knees.
Teacher holds child's hands as bent arms are swung strongly for-
    ward and upward, and child lifts his/her body clear of the box
    and lands in a semi squat on the mat. Later, child does the move
    alone.)

"Today we will try a 'Quick Squat' . . . "
(Child stands back from side of box, moves forward to Bunny Jump
    on to box, releases hands and jumps off.)
(Later, child brings feet through between hands, without feet touch-
    ing the box.)

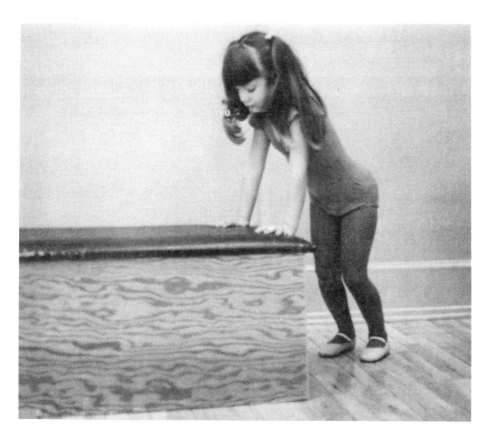

Figure 34. "Bunny jump onto the box."

BENCH

Benches may be purchased or constructed (see "Improvising Equipment" in Chapter X).

If a balance beam is built into the base, it becomes a very versatile piece of equipment.

The surface must be smooth and sliver free.

Mats must be placed where children will land.

Most low balance beam and low vaulting box activities can be adapted to the bench.

The following activities are unique to the bench.

> *"Let me see you waddle like a duck along the bench, then jump off...*
> *Can you walk on all fours like a monkey?...*

Can you walk like a bear?...
Now walk like an inch worm...
This time, slither like a seal..."
(Child lies on tummy at end of bench, reaches forward, grasps the sides, pulls body forward past hands; repeats to end.)

"Now pretend you are a dead bug..."
(Child lies on back, at end of bench, with feet up in the air, reaches back to grasp sides, pulls body along to end.)

"Sit on the bench, lift up your feet, and spin around to face the other end...
Now do it all the way around...
Lie on your tummy across the bench; now turn over to lie on your back...
Keep your body stretched..."

REUTER BOARD

The use of the reuter board with small children precedes mini-trampoline activities.

Have a landing mat in place with a chalk circle drawn where the children should land.

Teacher should hold the children's hands at first to give them confidence.

Some children will move swiftly through the following progressions; others may take months.

"Walk up the board, bounce three times, jump off and land low...
Walk up, bounce once and jump off...
Run up, bounce once and jump off...
Clap your hands while in the air...
Bend your knees and touch your feet while in the air...
Jump high in the air and turn to the side before you land...
     (¼ turn)
Jump high in the air and turn to the board before you land..."
     (½ turn)

Later add ¾ turn.

"Now when you land low, let me see you do a forward roll on the mat..."

Combinations:

Combine into a sequence.

Example: Walk up the board, bounce once and jump off, land low, forward roll, jump high in the air, balance on one foot to count three, bunny jump back to the end of the line for another turn.

LONG HANGING ROPES

Small children can develop upper-body strength through long hanging rope activities.

All attachments must be checked regularly.

Mats must be underneath the ropes.

If ropes are placed close together, all children swing in the same direction, at the same time.

To avoid discouragement, gentle swings are introduced before climbs.

> *"Can you hug the rope and go for a swing?...*
>
> *Pretend the mat is the river; can you swing across the river without getting your feet wet?...*
>
> *Now swing back again...*
>
> *Let me see you swing across the river and back, without resting on the other side?...*
>
> *Can you do this twice without getting your feet wet?..."*

Place a small cardboard box on the mat to make a rock.

> *"Can you swing across the river and not touch the rock?..."*

Repeat all of the above swings with the rock in place.

This makes the children raise their legs higher.

Raise the level of the rock by placing box on its end or by piling up two small boxes.

If children hit the cardboard boxes with their feet, they do not hurt themselves.

> *"Can you get your feet higher than your hands?...*
>
> *Come down gently...*
>
> *Can you swing gently with your feet higher than your hands?...*
>
> *Can you hug the rope with your hands and arms and feet?...*
>
> *Can you move your hands up the rope, then your feet?..."*

Make sure that you teach children to descend, hand under hand; *not slide* hands down, as rope burns will occur.

Place a ribbon halfway up the rope.

> *"Can you climb the rope to touch the ribbon and come down again, hand under hand, very slowly?*

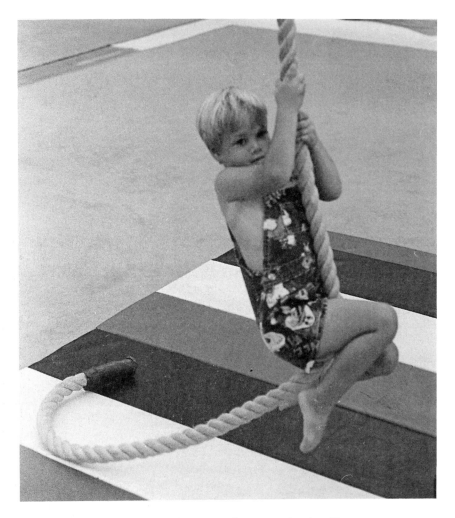

Figure 35. "Can you swing across the river?"

If you have two ropes close enough together, all swinging activities can be done using the two ropes.

Chapter V

DANCE ACTIVITIES

Dance is composed of the basic movements of life adapted to a rhythm, a theme, an idea, a stimulus, or an accompaniment.

It is a widely held belief that initially, all young boys and girls like to dance, to tap out a rhythm, to wiggle in time to music. It is only through bad experiences and adult comments, such as "It's sissy to dance," that boys get turned off dance. But, observe them as teenagers, responding to disco and rock music. Notice the amount of money spent on compact discs and tapes by preteens and teens.

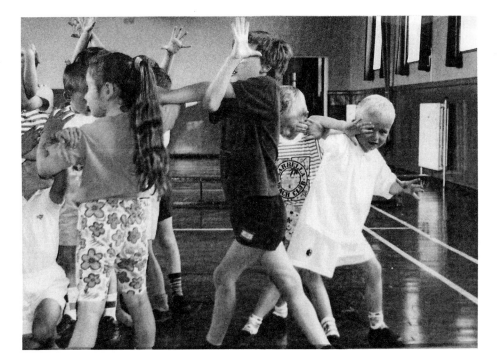

Figure 36. Young boys like to dance too.

Current research indicates that from birth through early childhood musical intelligence is evolving with concomitant changes in the brain. This development can be stimulated with rhythmic activities involving whole body movements. It is important that no children lose their early joy in moving to music and that adequate time be alloted to dance activities at all grade levels. The following is a program which has something for everyone. It is divided into two sections to show the two main approaches to teaching dance. A versatile teacher will intermingle activities from both sections to provide something of interest for all children; to give them the opportunity to be creative, to be exposed to other societies' dances, and to carry on their own culture's traditional dances. See Appendix B for a list of music resources for many of these dances which follow.

DANCE CHART

There are two main methods of teaching dance:

Creative: "Sow" Method
Teacher sows the seed of an idea for children to develop.

Traditional: "Show" Method
Teacher shows, children imitate.
The following program chart classifies dance activities according to the teaching method.

CREATIVE ("SOW" METHOD)	*TRADITIONAL* ("SHOW" METHOD)
Rhymes to move to	Icebreakers
Names to move to	Finger plays
Creative dance using rhythm instruments	Action songs
Creative dance using patterns	Singing games
Sounds to move to:	Folk dances
Body sounds	Ethnic dances
Sounds of nature	
Animal sounds	
Mechanical sounds	
Verses and poems	
Dance a story	
Hats, gloves, shoes, coats, dresses, wigs	
Pictures coming to life	

Statues
Sports
Shadows
Streamers and scarves

CREATIVE "SOW" METHOD ACTIVITIES

Rhymes To Move To

Objectives:

To develop a sense of rhythm.
To improve locomotor movements.
To stimulate rhyme-making by the children.
To give each child a personal rhyme.

Method:

Free spacing, facing teacher.
Teacher makes up rhymes for children in the class and suggests movements that fit the rhymes.
A few names are selected each day.
Children are then encouraged to make up their own rhymes for themselves, their classmates, and teacher.
The following are examples which a teacher could use by substituting names of children in his/her class.

"Jason, Jason is always chasing
I can too! I can too!"
(Children run around chasing each other; repeat a few times.)

"Lupe, Lupe jumped so high
She nearly hit her head on the sky."
(Children jump on the spot as high as they can.)

"Nancy, Nancy dances fancy
I can too! I can too!"
(Children dance any way they like.)

"Kelly, Kelly wobbles like jelly
I can too! I can too!"

"Enriqueta mails a letter
I can too! I can too!"

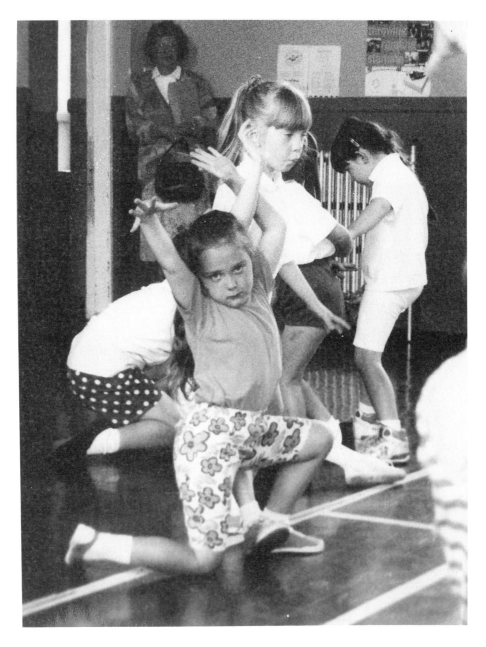

Figure 37. "Nancy, Nancy dances fancy."

"Leti, Leti wiggles like spaghetti
I can too! I can too!

"Toni, Toni rides on a pony
I can too! I can too!"

"George Soto snaps a photo
I can too! I can too!"

"Patrick Brown jumps up and down
I can too! I can too!"

"Randy, Randy, hops so dandy
I can too! I can too!"

Names To Move To

Objectives:

To develop a sense of rhythm.
To improve locomotor movements.
To give each child a moment as the center of attention.
To stimulate creative movement patterns.

Method:

Free spacing, facing teacher.
Teacher makes up movements to match the rhythm of the children's names.
Teacher and children move in a circle to rhythm of name, while owner of name stands in the middle.
Children are then encouraged to make up their own movement patterns.
The following are examples to give the teacher an idea of how a movement pattern can fit a name:

	Salvador Lopez	
"Sal-va-dor		*Lo-pez"*
run-run-run		jump-jump
	Maria Del Moro	
"Ma-ri-a		*Del-Mo-ro"*
run forward		run backward
swinging arms up		swinging arms down
	Jesus Figueroa	
"Je-sus		*Fig-uer-o-a"*
walk-walk		hop-hop-hop-hop
	El Paso, Texas	
"El-Pa-so		*Tex-as"*
run-run-run		leap-leap
	Portland, Oregon	
"Port-land		*O-re-gon"*
walk-walk		stomp-stomp-stomp

*United States of
America*

U-nit-ed-States-of   A-mer-i-ca"
skip-skip   jump and turn in air

Annabel Lee

"Ann-a-bel   Lee"
run-run-run   jump high and clap
                                                            hands high

Creative Dance Using Rhythm Instruments

Objectives:

To experience joy in dancing to own accompaniment.
To develop a sense of rhythm.
To improve locomotor movements.
To stimulate creative movement patterns.
To react to different sound qualities.

Accompaniments:

Piano
Music with catchy beat.
Rhythm instruments, either commercial or made by the children and
    teacher (see "Improvising Equipment" in Chapter X).
Instruments must make a sound, not necessarily a tune.
Children can decorate instruments using paints, felt pens, contact paper,
    felt, cutouts, Christmas bows and ribbons.
There must be no sharp edges, toxic paint, or harmful contents.
The instruments must be small enough for a young child to carry and
    play while "dancing."

Examples: Drums made from coffee cans, rolled oats containers, ice
cream buckets, fried chicken buckets, bleach containers.
Leave plastic lids on some containers to obtain a different sound.
Fill some with rice, gravel, or macaroni to develop as a shaker.
Decorate as an art project.
Shakers made from light bulbs (papier mâchéd), juice containers, alumi-
    num pie plates, margarine containers, plastic bleach bottles, egg-
    shaped pantyhose containers, two fan-shaped seashells, gourds.

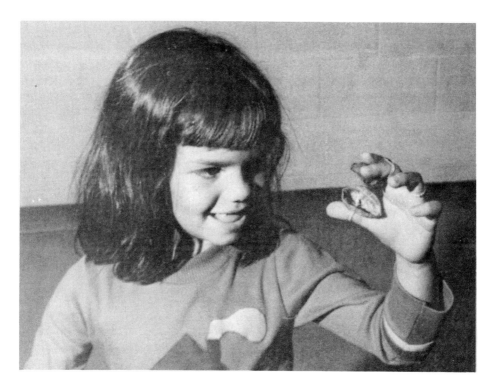

Figure 38. Finger castanets made from walnut shells.

Fill with different small items to obtain different sounds and decorate. Seal well to avoid spillages.

Tambourines made from two paper plates glued together; aluminum plates, single or double; two sour cream containers glued together.
Attach pop bottle tops, bells, or ribbons, and decorate.
Sticks made from mop handles, cut into 6″ lengths and decorated.
Coconut shell halves.
Cymbals, gongs, triangles, toy xylophones.
Old gloves, with bells or pop bottle caps sewn to the finger tips.
Old pots and wooden spoons.
Blocks of wood with elastic handles.
Banjo made with tissue box and rubber bands.
Wristlets or anklets: elastic with bells attached.
Finger castanets made from walnut shells.

Method:

To begin, teacher beats out a rhythm on a drum or another instrument. Children clap to time.

Repeat, with stamp, tap toes, walk, jump, hop, gallop, skip, etc.

Introduce change of level (high, medium, low).

Introduce change of force (light, medium, heavy).

Introduce change of direction (forward, backwards, sideways, diagonal).

Introduce change of size (large steps, little steps).

Children choose an instrument. Give them time to sound them (this will be very noisy).

Teacher puts on music or plays piano and asks children to keep time with their instruments, while sitting or kneeling facing the music source.

Teacher varies the rhythms: $4/4$, $2/4$, $6/8$, $3/4$, etc.

Children keep time at regular speed, half speed, double speed.

Child is chosen to "conduct" the class.

Class sits in circle, plays to record or piano, while two or three children "dance" around them.

They change places when tapped on shoulder.

Class sits in circle, plays to record or piano; one child is the Pied Piper who moves around outside of circle playing instrument for one circuit, taps another child on the shoulder to follow, until the whole class is up and moving, while playing instruments.

If the class is large, start with two or three Pied Pipers.

Groups take turns at playing instruments for other groups to dance.

Children play instruments unaccompanied by record or piano and dance any way they want to.

Children dance as the sound of their instrument suggests (light, heavy, slow, fast).

Teacher takes two or three contrasting instruments, asks the children to listen to the sound pattern he/she makes, and then move (dance) to that sound.

With Partner:

One child plays one or two instruments while the other dances.
Exchange roles.

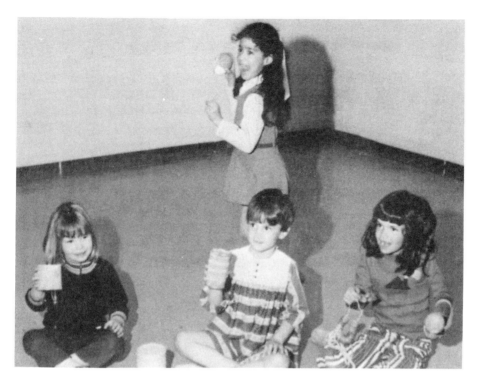

Figure 39. Class plays instruments while child is Pied Piper.

In Groups:

One or two children are the musicians and sit or kneel on the floor.
They decide on a sound pattern; other children in the group dance around them.
Several children are the musicians and decide on a sound pattern.
Other children are asked to do a dance that emphasizes a body part.

Examples: Elbow and knee dance.
Head and hand dance.
Tummy and hips dance.
Toes and fingers dance.
Wiggle-all-over dance.
At all times, teachers should encourage free, original movements.
Move around the class, praising, inciting, and helping.

Creative Dance Using Patterns

Objectives:

To stimulate creative movement patterns.
To awaken a desire to dance.
To improve locomotor movements.
To develop a sense of rhythm.
To develop awareness of directions.
To identify left and right.

Equipment:

Record player.
Records with catchy beat. Folk dance, "Cumberland Long Eight" is a useful record to do almost all basic dance steps to.

Method:

Free spacing, facing teacher and record player.
Start with an icebreaker to get the children moving (see "Icebreakers" in this Chapter).
Play "I like you, I don't like you."

> *"When I go like this* (beckon children forward),
> *it means I like you and I want you to jump towards me . . .*
> *When I go like this* (pretend to push children back),
> *it means I don't like you and I want you to jump backwards . . . "*

Put on record and beckon children forward for eight counts, push back for eight counts.
Repeat, using eight, four, two counts, until children are jumping wildly in all directions.
Change facial expressions from pleasure to displeasure as arm movements change.
Repeat, using walk, hop, skip, etc.
Play "Traffic Cops."

> *"When I point this way* (to left), *I want you to walk this way . . .*
> *When I point this way* (to right), *I want you to walk this way . . .*
> *Keep watching me, as I might change very suddenly . . . "*

Put on record and point to the left for eight counts . . . point to right for eight counts . . .

Repeat, using eight, four, two counts, until children are wiggling on the
  spot.

Repeat, using jump, hop, skip, gallop, etc.

This is also a good activity to introduce the slide, which is a gallop done
  sideways.

Repeat, using a child as the traffic cop.

Use Nursery Rhymes:

Teacher and children sing or recite the rhymes while they clap out the
  rhythm.

Teacher suggests movements that fit the rhymes.

Then the children are asked to fit the movements.

Examples:

"Baa baa black sheep, have you any wool?
(Walk, walk, walk, walk, run with little steps.)

Yes sir, yes sir, three bags full.
(Walk, walk, walk, walk, run with little steps.)

One for my master and one for my dame,
(Walk . . .)

And one for the little boy who lives down the lane."
(Run . . .)

Little Bo Peep
(Use skips, slides, gallops.)

Humpty Dumpty
(Use skips, slides, gallops.)

Little Jack Horner
(Use skips, jumps.)

Twinkle, Twinkle Little Star
(Use walks, claps, jumps.)

Making Patterns:

Teacher gives the children simple movement patterns.

These may be done to music or unaccompanied.

Examples:

Four walks forward, four walks backwards, eight jumps on the spot, with
  hand claps.

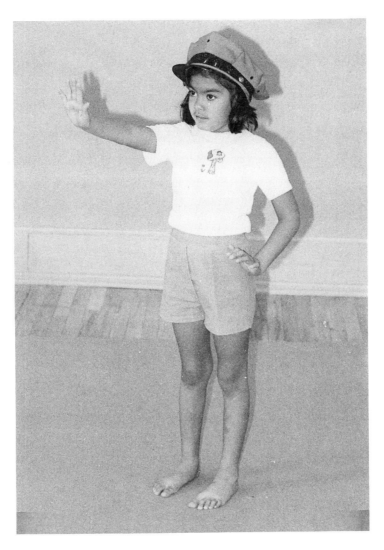

Figure 40. Traffic Cop.

Eight slides to the right, eight slides to the left (indicate direction with
arms). eight gallops to the right, eight gallops to the left.

Four slides to the right, four slides to the left, two slides to the right, two
slides to the left, one slide to the right, left, right, left.

Four gallops to the right, four gallops to the left, four skips forward, four
skips backwards.

Four gallops to the right, four gallops to the left, four skips towards
teacher, four skips away from teacher, eight skips in a circle.

Add claps, snaps, hand waves, and hip slaps to above patterns.

Up to now, the teacher has been providing the patterns.

Now ask the children to make up their very own "dances" to the same music.

At first, limit them to using walks and jumps only, or walks and skips, skips and slides, gallops, skips and claps, etc.

Then let them choose any steps for their "dances."

Have half the class watch while the other half shows their "dances," and vice versa.

Choose one simple dance for the whole class to copy.

After class, help the child whose dance was chosen to write it up in a large book made of butcher paper and to illustrate it on the opposite page.

Let the child give the dance a title, such as "Danny's Dance," "Gina's Jig," "Peter's Polka," "Lupe's Lilt."

Put the book on the class library shelf for free reading and add to it during the semester until each child has a dance included.

This same approach can be used for the children to work with a partner and in threes, or fours.

Larger groups are too difficult for young children.

After a folk dance tune has been used for pattern making, teach the real folk dance.

Sounds To Move To

Objectives:

To stimulate creative movement.
To tune in to sound differences and to respond with movements.
To exercise the whole body.

Method:

Free spacing, facing teacher.

Body Sounds:

> *"Today I am going to give you two different laughs.*
> *I want you to make up movements that fit them . . .*
> *Ho! Ho! Ho! . . . Hee! Hee! Hee! . . . "*

Give the children time to experiment.

Encourage children to use their own sound accompaniment.

Do not demonstrate unless there is no response.

Draw attention to different interpretations.

Repeat, using other sounds such as sneeze, hiccup, cough, clap, click, chatter, sigh, yawn, buzz, hiss.

Ask children to make up combinations of these sounds and to interpret them with movements.

Let half the class watch, while the other half performs.

Sounds of Nature: Use the above approach, using sounds such as the sea (waves lapping, breaking on the shore), a waterfall, thunder, rain, wind, a fire crackling.

Animal Sounds: Zoo, farm, jungle animals, sea creatures, birds, insects.

Children will copy the animal's movements as they make the sound.

This is to be encouraged.

Draw attention to the different ways the animals move.

Mechanical Sounds: Car, motorcycle, truck, bus, train, small plane, jet, helicopter, ambulance, fire truck, tractor, lawn mower, lawn sprinkler, washing machine, blender, ice maker, cake mixer. Children will imitate the action of the vehicle or machine.

Verses and Poems

Objectives:

To interpret a verse or poem through movement.

To awaken an appreciation for poetry.

To stimulate original interpretations.

To exercise the whole body.

Equipment:

Verses or poems that lend themselves to being interpreted in movement and are suitable for the age group.

Method:

Free spacing, facing teacher.

> *"Today I'm going to recite you a verse and then we're going to do what it says . . ."*

Teacher recites the verse, with expression, and does the actions to match.

Children will start to copy him/her.

"Now you have to help me say the verse, and we'll all do what the verse says . . . "

Recite the verse slowly, giving time for the actions.

When the children have got the idea, teacher just recites the verse and does not impose the actions.

Children are asked to do what the verse says.

The following verses have been used with success by many teachers:

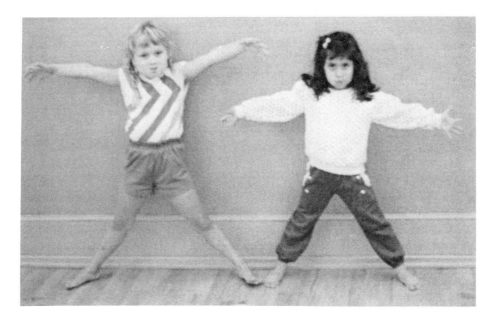

Figure 41. "Make yourself as fat as a cat."

Make yourself as tall as a house
Make yourself as small as a mouse
Make yourself as thin as a pin
Make yourself as fat as a cat

Small as a mouse
Tall as a tree
Wide as a house
Now spin like me

Up I stretch on tippy toe
Down to touch my heels I go
Up again my arms I send
Down again my knees I bend

I can run and I can hop
I can spin 'round like a top
I can stretch my arms out wide
As I slide from side to side

To and fro, to and fro
Sweeping with my broom I go
All the fallen leaves I sweep
In a big and tidy heap

Mix a pancake
Stir a pancake
Pop it in the pan
Fry the pancake
Toss the pancake
Catch it if you can!

I am a giant who stamps his feet
I am a little elf, small and neat
I am a little mouse curled up small
And I'm a great big bouncing ball

I clap up high
I clap down low
I jump, jump, jump
And down I go

I can climb like a monkey at the zoo
I can jump like a jolly kangaroo
I can squat like a big green frog
I can run as fast as my dog

Stepping over stepping stones
one, two, three
Stepping over stepping stones
come with me!
The river's very fast, and the
river's very wide
And we'll step across on stepping
stones
To reach the other side
My little puppy's name is Rags
He eats so much that his tummy sags
His ears flip flop, his tail wig wags
And when he walks, he zigs and zags

See me gallop down the street
See how I can stamp my feet
Now I stop and paw the ground
Listen! I don't make a sound
Now I kick my heels up high
Whoever saw a horse so spry

Little Arabella Miller
Found a wooly caterpillar
First it crawled upon her mother
Then upon her baby brother
All said, "Arabella Miller
Take away that caterpillar!"

Last evening cousin Peter came
Last evening cousin Peter came
Last evening cousin Peter came
To say that he was here
He hung his hat upon a peg
He hung his hat upon a peg
He hung his hat upon a peg
To show that he was here
He wiped his shoes upon the mat, etc.
He kicked his shoes off one by one, etc.
He danced about in his stockinged feet,
  etc.
He played he was a great big bear, etc.
He tossed us up into the air, etc.
He made a bow and said, "Goodbye," etc.

If I were a little bird, high up in the sky,
This is how I'd flap my wings and fly, fly, fly.

If I were a friendly dog, going for a run,
This is how I'd wag my tail when having fun.

If I were a cat I'd sit by the fireplace,
This is how I'd use my paws to wash my face.

If I were an elephant, very big and strong.
This is how I'd wave my trunk and walk along.

If I were a kangaroo, I would leap and bound,
This is how I'd jump and jump all around.

If I were a camel tall, slowly I would stride.
This is how I'd rock and sway from side to side.

If I were a tall giraffe, living in the zoo.
This is how I'd bend my neck and look at you.

To introduce a poem, the teacher reads or recites and points out that it is telling the children something.

Teacher rereads the poem, encouraging the children to listen carefully and to think how they could do what the poem says.

Draw attention to action words, mood, atmosphere, etc.

Teacher asks the children to find their very own space.

(S)he reads the poem with expression, while they interpret it in movement.

The following poems lend themselves to free interpretation:

"Some One"—Walter De La Mere
"Softly, Drowsily"—Walter De La Mere
"Feet"—Myra Cohn Livingston
"Song of the Train"—David McCord
"The White Window"—James Stephens
"Little Snail"—Hilda Conkling
"Duck's Ditty"—Kenneth Grahame
"Hiawatha's Childhood"—H.W. Longfellow
"First Snow"—Marie Louise Allen
"Galoshes"—Rhoda Bacmeister
"Furry Bear"—A.A. Milne
"The Gingerbread Man"—Rowena Bennett
"Mice"—Rose Fyleman
"On Our Way"—Eve Merriam
"The Swing"—Robert Louis Stevenson
"Holding Hands"—Lenore M. Link
"My Zipper Suit"—Marie Louise Allen
"Jump or Jiggle"—Evelyn Beyer
"Cats"—Mary Britton Miller
"Fog"—Carl Sandburg

Dance A Story

Objectives:

To interpret a story through movement.
To stimulate original interpretations.

Equipment:

Stories that are read to class, preferably with opportunities for a lot of action.

Examples: "The Tale of Peter Rabbit"
"The Three Billy Goats Gruff"
"The Little Engine That Could."
"Mike Mulligan and His Steam Shovel"
"Millions of Cats"
"Dr. Seuss Stories"
"The Sleeping Beauty"
"Goldilocks and the Three Bears"
"Cinderella"
"Peter Pan"
"Little Red Riding Hood"
"Aesop's Fables"
"Andersen's Fairy Tales"
"What Do You Want to Be?"—Richard Scarry
"Who Said Boo?"—Cass Hollander
"Mirror, Look! Mirror Do!"—Cecelia Avalos
"The Popcorn Popper"—Joanne Nelson

Method:

Teacher reads the story to the class, then tells them that they are going to "play" the story.

(S)he paraphrases the story, while the class acts out all the characters with a minimum of direction.

Another approach is for the teacher to choose children for the principal characters of a story and to have the other children form such things as trees in the forest, wind rushing by, carriages of a train, tunnels, hills, castle, etc.

Make sure that all children have a principal role at some time.

Aim for whole body movement interpretations rather than miming.

Have children make up a story for the class to interpret.

Hats[1]

Objectives:

To stimulate creative movement.
To develop a sense of rhythm.
To improve locomotor movements.

---

[1]Reprinted from *Instructor,* February 1974. Copyright© 1974 by the Instructor Publications, Inc. Reprinted by permission of Scholastic, Inc.

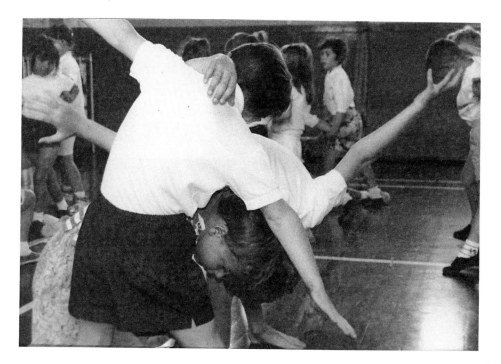

Figure 42. Encourage free original movements.

Equipment:

A collection of hats preferably washable or disposable (such as worn by a cook, painter, sailor, swimmer, skier, jockey, farmer, fast food worker); a fashion hat, baby's bonnet, ear muffs, tiara, crown, Santa Claus hat; head gear made by children (such as rabbit ears, Easter bonnet, Indian headdress, witch's hat).

Music with a catchy tune.

Method:

Children sit in a circle, with hats piled in the middle.

Teacher chooses one or two children to put on hats and to stand outside the circle.

> *"When I play the music, I want you to move around the circle and pretend to be the owner of the hat...*
> *The rest of you will clap in time with the music..."*

When the children have gone around once, stop the music, tell them to return the hats to the center of the circle, and to tap another child on the shoulder to go choose a hat.

If there are enough hats for all the children, let them choose one each and play the music for them to move.

When the music stops, they exchange hats.

When the music starts, they move again, like the original hat owner would move.

The above approach can also be used with other clothes such as gloves, shoes, scarves, coats, dresses, wigs.

More time would need to be given to get dressed and undressed.

Pictures Coming To Life

Objectives:

To stimulate creative movement.
To develop an awareness of art.

Equipment:

Pictures, paintings, photographs, posters.
Record player and records (optional).
Large wooden frame or lines drawn on wall.

Method:

Children sit facing the teacher.

> *"Today, I have a picture to show you...*
> *It was painted a long time ago by a very famous man called Degas... "*
> (Teacher shows Degas painting of ballet dancers.)

> *"Look very carefully and see what the people in the picture are doing...*
> *How many people are there?...*
> *Do you think three of you could make that picture with your bodies?... "*
> (Choose three children and help them take the formation in the frame.)

> *"Now when I play the music, I want you to come to life and dance like the people in the picture...*
> *You may step out of the frame and dance in this space... "*

Repeat, using different pictures and different children.
Do not allow the other children to sit too long.

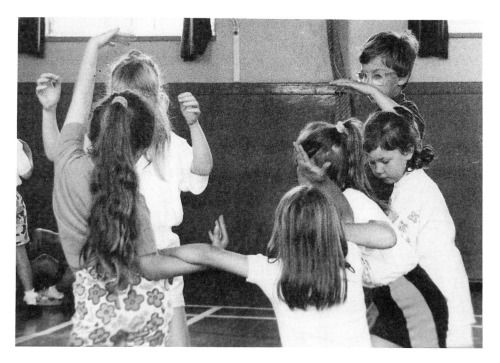

Figure 43. "When the music starts, dance like the people in the picture."

Statues

Objectives:

To stimulate original interpretations.
To develop a sense of rhythm.
To improve locomotor movements and balance.

Equipment:

Statues or pictures.
Music with a catchy beat, drum, or piano.

Method:

Free spacing, facing the teacher and the music source.
Teacher shows the children statues or pictures and discusses what they
   are and how still they are.

"Today we are going to play at being statues...

I will play some music for you to walk to...

When the music stops, I want you to make yourself into a statue of an animal...

You must keep very still until the music starts again..."

Repeat, using other statues such as dancers, sportsmen, pioneers, kings, and queens, etc.

Use other locomotor movements.

Sometimes, let the children make a statue for the other children and teacher to guess what it is.

With Partner:

Repeat the above activities with a partner.

This will require cooperation to remain very still.

It usually results in a more complex interpretation.

In Groups:

Repeat the above activities.

Another approach is to have the children take the form of a statue, to come to life when the music starts, and to freeze when the music stops.

This can also be done without accompaniment.

Sports

Objectives:

To encourage creative movement.

To develop an awareness of sports actions.

Equipment:

Sports pictures or statues.

Music (optional).

Method:

Free spacing, facing the teacher.

> *"Today we are going to pretend we are playing a sport (or game)...*
> *Look at the men in this picture and tell me what sport they are playing..."*

(Show a baseball picture.)

> *"Now when I play the music, let's all pretend to be baseball players...*
> *What sort of movements will we be doing?...throwing...pitching...*
> *hitting...*
> *catching...fielding...running bases."*

Give the children time to experiment.

Do not demonstrate unless there is no response.

Move around to encourage, incite, and help.

Repeat, using football, basketball, volleyball, tennis, hockey, soccer, etc.

Shadows

Objectives:

To stimulate creative movement patterns.

To develop an awareness of size and shape.

Equipment:

Music, drum, or tambourine (these are optional).

This activity may also be done without accompaniment.

Method:

Line formation, facing a wall, on a sunny day.

> *"Today it is sunny and we all have a shadow...*
> *When I play the music I want you to make your shadow dance..."*

Play music of different tempos to encourage different movement qualities.

Use the same approach, but encourage children to make their shadows
    tall, small, fat, thin, wobbly, wiggly, very still, etc.

Children join up with a partner to make their combined shadows dance,
    make animal shapes, machines, trees, etc.

One child dances while partner moves behind like a shadow.

In Groups:

Children join hands to make a line of paper dolls.
Teacher gives the command to raise, lower arms, kick legs, bend knees, nod heads, rock from side to side, etc., in unison.
Children make up their own routines.

Streamers and Scarves

Objectives:

To stimulate creative movement.
To introduce focus.
To exercise the whole body but particularly the upper body.
To emphasize prepositions.

Equipment:

Streamers, ribbons on sticks, one for each child (see "Improvising Equipment" in Chapter X).
Nylon scarves.
Music.
This activity may also be done without accompaniment.

Method:

Free spacing, facing the teacher, with room to move without bumping into each other.

> *"Today we are going to make our streamers (scarves) dance while we dance...*
> *Give yourselves plenty of room and see if you can make your streamers do what mine is doing..."*

Make circles in front of the body, at sides, overhead.
Change hands.
Repeat, using figure eights, arcs, spirals, serpents (big vertical waves), snakes (small horizontal waves on the ground), free forms.

> *"Now I want you to make your streamers do something different...*
> *Make them go high... low... in front of you... behind you... under you...*
> *Make them go fast... then slow...*
> *Now can you walk around and make your streamers dance beside... behind... above... in front of you..."*

Repeat, using skip, gallop, run, dance.

Repeat, using kneel, sit, lie.

Encourage a change of hands.

Maintain good spacing.

Give children two scarves and ask them to pretend they have butterfly wings.

TRADITIONAL "SHOW" METHOD ACTIVITIES

Icebreaker

This traditional activity is presented first at the beginning of any dance class to get the children moving.

Objectives:

To give some direction to the children's movements.

To develop listening skills.

To awaken a sense of rhythm.

To improve locomotor movements.

To introduce dance steps.

Equipment:

Music with catchy beat.

Method:

Sitting: Ask the children to sit on the floor, facing the teacher and the record player.

Teacher also sits on the floor.

Everyone cups their hands behind their ears (make big elephant ears), listens to the music, picks up the beat, and claps in time with the teacher and the music.

Teacher leads the group with hand claps, reaching high, low, forward and backwards, in a circle, in the air catching bugs; finger snaps (one and two hands), head nods (yes and no), eyebrows raising (dancing), winking (one and two eyes), nose wiggles, ear wiggles, arm flaps (like wings), waving to teacher (one and two hands), bumps (seats on floor), kicking legs in the air, toe taps on the floor (one, both, alternate).

Standing: Everyone stands in place and in time with the teacher and the music, do such movements as high kicks (forward, backwards, sideways), toe taps on the floor (waking up earthworms or the downstairs neighbors), hip wiggles, jumps (bouncing like a ball), hops, knee dips, turnarounds.
Follow Me: Teacher, or the child leader, moves around the room with the other children following, copying his/her movements.
They walk (big and small, high and low, stomp, march), jump, hop, gallop, skip, slide, leap, dance freely, etc.
Change level, direction, force, speed, size, emotion, or character.

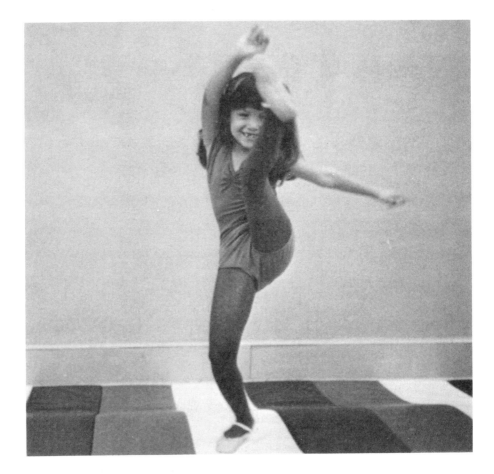

Figure 44. Ice breaker: high kicks.

Teacher leads the group back to the starting point, sits down, and finishes with claps only, in time to the music.

If more suitable, the children return to the starting point, but remain standing, in order to go straight into the next activity.

The icebreaker can also be used to present traditional body exercises in a more fun manner.

Finger Plays[2]

Objective:

To enjoy an activity when space is limited and/or when weather is inclement.

Method:

Children sit on the floor, facing the teacher.
Teacher recites a verse and does the actions.
Children copy.

Examples:

Fee fie foe fum	Point to each finger
See my finger	Point to index finger
See my thumb	Point to thumb
Fee fie foe fum	Point to each finger again
Finger's gone	Hide finger in fist
So is thumb	Hide thumb
Here is Mother Robin	Point to thumb
Here's the apple tree	Point to index finger
Where she keeps her children	
There are one, two, three	Count last three fingers
Way up in the apple tree	Point upward with index finger
Two little apples smiled down at me	Hold up two fingers
I shook that tree as hard as I could	Make shaking motions with hands and arms
And down came those apples	Hands sweep down and open wide
MMMMMM! Were they good	Rub stomach
Tap at the door	Tap one hand with fingers of other
Peek in	Form fingers into rings around eyes
Turn the knob	Make turning motion with other hand
Walk in	Walk fingers of one hand up opposite arm
And—shut the door	Clap loudly

---

[2]Verses reprinted from *Motor Development in the Preschool Years,* Louise Skinner, Charles C Thomas, 1979.

Five little monkeys	Hold up five fingers
Jumping on a bed	Wiggle fingers up and down
One fell off	
And cracked his head	Tap head with knuckles
He ran to the doctor	Move arms in running motion
And the doctor said,	
"That's what you get	Shake index finger
For jumping on the bed."	
Repeat with four, three, two, one	

Kitty, kitty, kitty, kitty	Extend one hand, palm up,
All my little ones so pretty	and beckon with index finger
You and you and you and you,	Point to four children
Let me hear how you can mew	
Mew, mew, mew, mew	Children mew

Action Songs

Objectives:

To introduce traditional action songs.
To develop a sense of rhythm.
To exercise the whole body.

Equipment:

Record player and records, or piano accompaniment.

Method:

Free spacing, unless specified in an individual action song.
(Note: Actions are dictated by the words. Teacher leads and the children
   follow.)

Bouncing Ball

"See how I can bounce my ball
Never, never let it fall
One and two and three and four
Hold it tight and sit on the floor.

See how I throw up my ball
Never, never let it fall
One and two and three and four
Hold it tight and stand up tall."

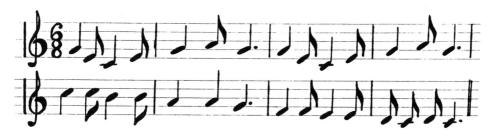

Figure 45. Music for "Bouncing Ball."

Digging

"Digging, digging with my spade
See the great big hole I've made
Now I build a castle high
Right up to the bright blue sky.

Digging, digging, with my spade,
See the great big hole I've made
Now I'll jump across and back
And run right round and round the track."

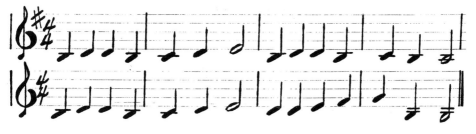

Figure 46. Music for "Digging."

Windmill

"If I had a windmill, a windmill, a windmill
If I had a windmill, I know what I'd have it do.

I'd have it draw the water, the water, the water
I'd have it draw the water, up from the river below.

I'd have it make a duck pond, a duck pond, a duck pond
I'd have it make a duck pond, so ducks and geese could swim.

The ducks would make their wings flap, their wings flap,
their wings flap
The ducks would make their wings flap, and then they would
say, "Quack, Quack!"

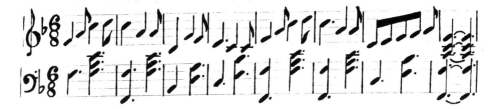

Figure 47. Music for "Windmill."

The geese would stretch their necks up, their necks up, their necks up,
The geese would stretch their necks up, and then they would say,
"SS–SS."

Teapot

"I'm a little teapot short and stout,
Here is my handle; here is my spout.
When I get all steamed up then I shout,
Just tip me over; pour me out."

Baby Ducks

"Have you seen the baby ducks waddling to the water?
Mother, father, baby ducks, grandmama and daughter."
(All waddle in line, when name is called Mother
stands up, father stretches tall, baby ducks squat,
grandmama wobbles from side to side, daughter
jumps up and down.)

"Have you seen them flap their wings floating on the water?
Mother, father, etc . . .

Have you seen them dip their bills drinking in the water?
Mother, father, etc . . .

Have you seen them stretch their necks, swimming in the water?
Mother, father, etc . . .

Have you seen them going home, waddling from the water?
Mother, father, etc.

Singing Games

Objectives:

To introduce traditional singing games.
To provide a lead into folk dance.
To develop a sense of rhythm,
To exercise the whole body.

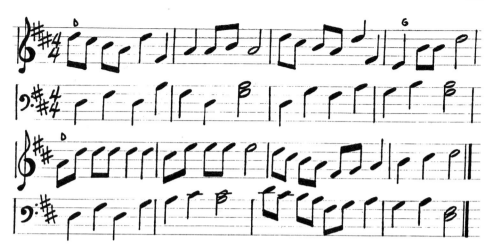

Figure 48. Music for "Teapot."

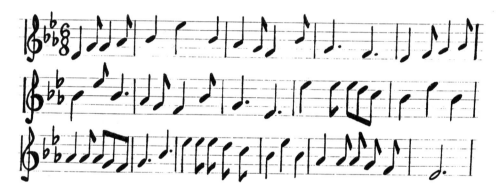

Figure 49. Music for "Baby Ducks."

Equipment:

Record player, records, or piano accompaniment (optional).

Method:

Formations are specified for each singing game.
Teacher stands where all the children can see and hear him/her.

Hammers

Children sit in a circle, with one child in the middle.
Their legs are stretched out in front of them, and their hands are
  clenched to form hammers.

Children sing a verse to the child in the middle, who does the actions. All sing and do the actions to the chorus.

> *"Billy hammers with one hammer, one hammer, one hammer*
> *Billy hammers with one hammer, this fine day."*
> (Child in center taps ground with right fist.)
> Chorus:

> *"We all hammer with one hammer, one hammer, one hammer*
> *We all hammer with one hammer, this fine day."*
> (All tap the ground with right fists.)

> *"Billy hammers with two hammers, two hammers, two hammers*
> *Billy hammers with two hammers, this fine day."*
> (Child in center taps the ground with right and left fists.)
> Chorus:

> *"We all hammer with two hammers, etc. . . . "*
> (All tap the ground with right and left fists.)

Repeat, using:

Three hammers (2 fists and right heel).

Four hammers (2 fists and 2 heels).

Five hammers (2 fists, 2 heels, head nods).

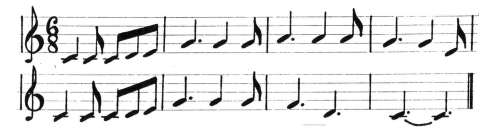

Figure 50. Music for "Hammers."

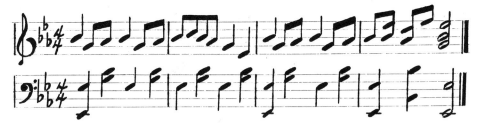

Figure 51. Music for "Punchinello."

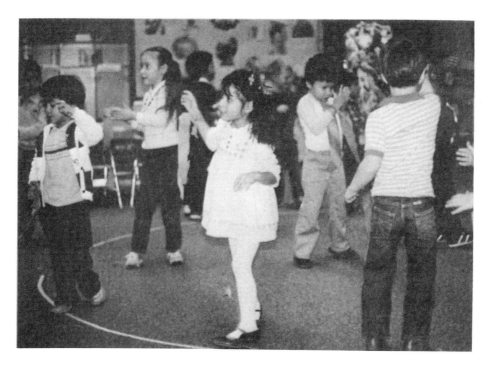

Figure 52. "We'll do it too, Punchinello funny fellow."

Punchinello

Children stand in a single circle, ready to move to the right.
One child, "Punchinello," stands in the center, ready to lead the movements.

> *"Look who is here, Punchinello, funny fellow,*
> *Look who is here, Punchinello, funny man."*
> (Children walk, run, skip around in a circle, singing to the child standing in the center.)

> *"What can you do, Punchinello, funny fellow?*
> *What can you do, Punchinello, funny man?*
> (Children stand still and shake index finger at the child in the center who does an exercise, animal move, etc.)

> *"We'll do it too, Punchinello, funny fellow,*
> *We'll do it too, Punchinello, funny man."*
> (Children copy movements of child in the center.)

"Whom do you choose, Punchinello, funny fellow?
Whom do you choose, Punchinello, funny man?"

(Children walk around in a circle again; child in center closes eyes, points to the circle, and pivots around. On "man," whomever is pointed at becomes Punchinello.)

The Little Mice Are Creeping

Children kneel on the floor in a designated area.
One child, "cat," stands off to the side.

"The little mice are creeping, creeping, creeping.
The little mice are creeping, all around the house."

(Children sing and creep around the space.)

"The little mice are eating, eating, eating
The little mice are eating, all around the house."

(Children stop and pretend to eat.)

"The little mice are sleeping, sleeping, sleeping.
The little mice are sleeping, all around the house."

(Children curl up and sleep.)

The big grey cat is creeping, creeping, creeping
The big grey cat is creeping, all around the house.

("Cat" walks slowly, quietly, through the sleeping mice.)

The little mice are running, running, running.
The little mice are running, all around the house."

(Mice wake up and scurry around, while the cat tries to tag them.)

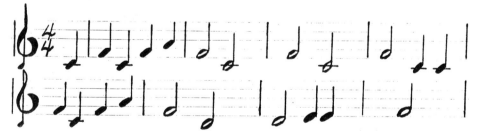

Figure 53. Music for "The Little Mice Are Creeping."

My Pigeon House

Boys stand close together in a single circle, with hands joined, to make a
  pigeon house.
Girls squat in the middle (pigeons).

> *"My pigeon house I open wide to set my pigeons free."*
> (Boys step back and raise arms; pigeons fly out through spaces and
>   fly around outside.)
>
> *"They fly all around in merry flight, and light on the tallest tree."*
> (On "tree," pigeons stand behind the boys, who have stretched their
>   arms very high.)
>
> *"And when they return from their merry flight."*
> (Pigeons fly back to the center of the circle.)
>
> *"I shut the doors and say, 'goodnight,'"*
> (Boys lower their arms and move in close to cover the pigeons.)
>
> *"Coo-oo, Coo-oo, Coo-oo, Coo-oo, Coo-oo, Coo-oo, Coo-oo."*
> (Everyone keeps very still while pigeons "Coo."

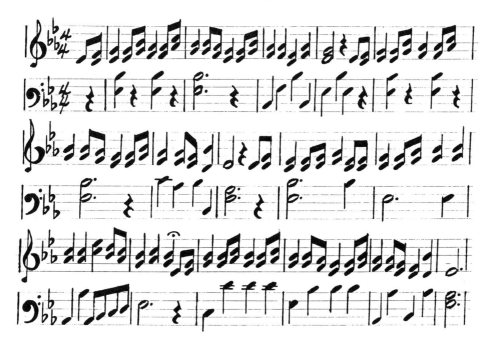

Figure 54. Music for "My Pigeon House."

The Thread Follows The Needle

Children stand in lines of five, with the first child touching the wall. Hands are joined to form a "thread."

> *"The thread follows the needle,*
> *The thread follows the needle,*
> *In and out the needle goes,*
> *While mother mends the children's clothes."*

(Last child in line, the "needle," leads the other children under the arm of the child nearest the wall. (S)he turns in place, to finish with arms crossed, but still touching the wall with one hand.)

The words and actions are repeated as the "needle" leads the thread through the next arch, and the second child turns in place to finish with arms crossed.

These actions are repeated until all the arches have been gone through and all the children are joined up with arms crossed.

On a signal from the music, all the children raise their held hands, turn towards the wall, and unwind the thread.

Alley, Alley, Oo

Formation is the same as for "The Thread Follows The Needle."

> *"The good ship sails through the alley alley oo,*
> *The alley alley oo, the alley alley oo,*
> *The good ship sails through the alley alley oo,*
> *On the nineteenth of December."*

Actions are the same as for "The Thread Follows The Needle" until the last chorus. While this is sung, the children move backwards and inwards to join up into a circle.

All have arms crossed and are facing outwards.

All jump up and down, while they recite:

> *"Jump, jump, sugar lump*
> *All the ladies in a bump!"*

(Then they all raise their held hands and turn inwards to unfold arms.)

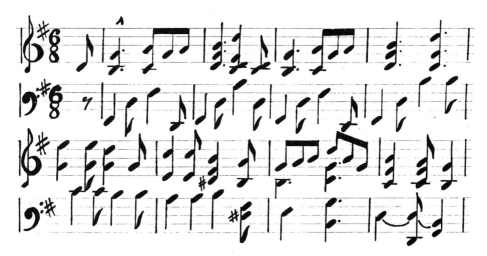

Figure 55. Music for "The Thread Follows The Needle." Courtesy of A.S. Barnes and Company.

A Tiny Little Woman

Children are in pairs, facing each other, in a double circle.

"A tiny little woman, and a tiny little man."
(Girl squats down, while the boy presses her gently on the shoulder;
  then she comes up, while the boy squats down.)

"A tiny little kettle and a tiny little pan."
(Repeat the above actions.)

"You take the kettle and I'll take the pan."
(Both point at each other, then point at themselves.)

"Said the tiny little woman to the tiny little man."
(Repeat the first actions.)

Lubin Loo

Children are in a single circle, hands joined, ready to move to the
  right.
Slide, skip, etc.
Chorus:

"Here we go Lubin Loo, here we go Lubin light,
Here we go Lubin Loo, all on a Saturday night."
(All slide to the right.)

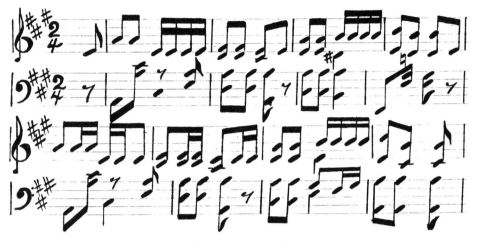

Figure 56. Music for "A Tiny Little Woman."

*"I put my right hand in, I put my right hand out,
I shake it a little, a little, and turn myself about."*
(Children stand still and put their right hands into the circle, then
    out, then shake them vigorously, and turn around.)

Chorus is repeated between each verse.
Verses are repeated with the left hand, right foot, left foot, head, and
    whole self.
On "whole self," children jump in and out.

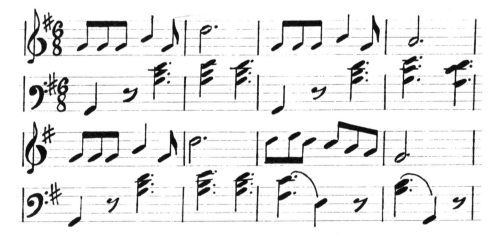

Figure 57. Music for "Lubin Loo." Courtesy of Bell and Hyman, Publisher.

Market Gate

Partners are in a double circle, elbows linked.

> *"When my father goes with mother to the market gate."*
> (Partners walk in a circle, counterclockwise.)

> *"Oh yes, yes so."*
> (Partners face each other, clap their own hands to the right and the
>   left, nod their heads to the right and the left.)

> *"They do not come back home until the evening late.*
> *Oh yes, yes so."*
> (Repeat the above actions.)

> *"Fie-de-re, fi-de-ra, fi-de-re-ra-ra."*
> (Partners join hands, do three skips around on the spot.
> On "ra-ra," they clap hands twice.)

> *"Fie-de-re, fi-de-ra, fi-de-re-ra-ra."*
> (Repeat the above actions.)

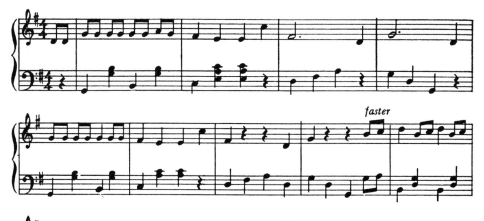

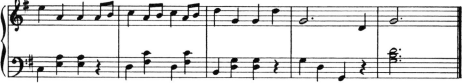

Figure 58. Music for "Market Gate." Courtesy of Department of Public Instruction, Queensland, Australia.

"Oh yes, yes so."
(Partners step to the right, bow or curtsy.
Repeat to the left.)

I See A Tiny Little Cottage

Children are in a single circle.

"I see a tiny little cottage,"
(All skip, slide, walk, etc., counterclockwise.)

"With a jolly pointed roof like that."
(All stand still and raise arms to make a pointed roof.)

"I see a tiny little cottage,
With a pointed roof like that."
(Repeat the above actions.)

"Around the cottage is a garden."
(All slide counterclockwise.)

"With a hedge so low, so low like that."
(All squat down to make a low hedge with hands.)

"Around the cottage is a garden.
With a hedge so low like that."
(Repeat the above actions.)

"And in the garden trees are swaying."
(Raise arms and sway from side to side.)

"And calling little birds like that."
(All fly around themselves.)

"And in the garden trees are swaying.
And calling birds like that."
(Repeat the above actions.)

"Ten dancing children make a circle."
(All skip counterclockwise with hands joined.)

"And then sit on the lawn like that."
(All drop hands and sit crosslegged.)

"Ten dancing children make a circle.
And then sit down like that."
(Repeat the above actions.)

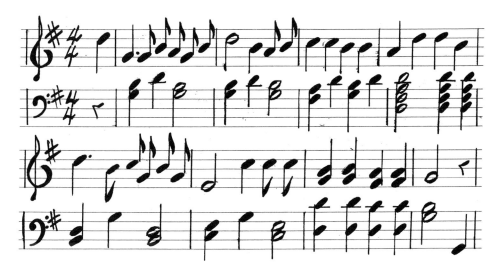

Figure 59. Music for "I See a Tiny Little Cottage."

Folk Dances

Objectives:

To introduce traditional folk dances.
To foster cross-cultural activities.
To experience enjoyment of folk dancing.
To improve locomotor movements.
To introduce basic dance steps.

Equipment:

Record player, records, tapes.
Sashes or cummerbunds to distinguish partners.

Method:

Formations are specified for each folk dance.
Make sure that all children are involved.
If one child is left over, have a threesome dance together.
Teacher stands where all the children can see and hear him/her.

La Raspa (Mexico)

Formation:

Double circle, partners facing, hands on hips.

Steps:

Bleking (spring left, place right heel forward, repeat to right, then left, then right).

Movements:

Start with left foot, four blekings.

Join right elbow with partner, hold left arm overhead, eight skips around each other.

Repeat, with left elbows joined, in the other direction.

Skip Annika (Sweden)

Formation:

Double circle, partners side by side, facing counterclockwise.

Inside hands are joined; outside hands are on hips.

Steps:

Walk, skip.

Movements:

Four slow walks forward, turn and bow to partner.

Repeat.

Sixteen fast walks forward, swinging inside arms.

Sixteen fast skips forward, finish facing partner.

Stamp the left foot forward, clap own hands.

Stamp the right foot backward, clap own hands.

Slap hips, clap own hands, clap partner's hands three times, very quickly.

Repeat the second movement.

Sixteen fast skips forward, swinging inside arms.

Repeat the whole dance.

La Vinca (Italy)

Formation:

Double circle, partners facing, hands joined.

Steps:

Slide, stamp, run.

Movements:

Sixteen fast slides counterclockwise.
Release hands, stamp feet three times.
Clap hands three times (one clap low, one clap medium, one clap high).
Shake index finger at partner three times.
Turn around self with three small runs.
Repeat the second movement.
Repeat the whole dance.

Seven Jumps (Denmark)

Formation:

Single circle, facing center, hands joined.

Steps:

Walk or run, step kicks sideways.

Movements:

Seven runs counterclockwise, stamp left foot.
Seven runs clockwise, stamp right foot.
Starting left, eight step kicks sideways.
On chord, kneel down on one knee, get up very quickly.
Repeat the above.
Each time a chord is added, the children add one of the following
    movements:
Kneel on two knees.
Put right elbow on floor.
Put left elbow on floor.
Put right fist on floor.
Put left fist on floor.
Put forehead on floor (or forward roll and spring high in the air).

Clap Dance (Germany)

Formation:

Double circle, partners facing, hands on hips.

Step:

Slide.

Movements:

Slap hips, clap own hands, clap partner's right hand.
Repeat with left hand.
Repeat, clap right and left hands quickly.
Repeat, clap partner's two hands.
Join hands with partner.
Eight fast slides counterclockwise.
Eight fast slides clockwise.
Repeat the whole dance.
To change partners, on the last two slides, the girl moves down to the
    next boy.

Troika (Russia)

Formation:

Children in lines of three in a circle, hands joined, facing counterclockwise.

Step:

Run.

Movements:

Four runs forward to diagonal right.
Four runs forward to diagonal left.
Repeat to the right and the left.
Children raise arms to form arches.
Right child runs under left arch.
Left child runs under right arch.

Center child turns under arch each time and runs on the spot.
Children join hands in a triangle.
Twelve runs, clockwise.
Stamp feet, left, right, left, hold.
Twelve runs, counterclockwise.
Stamp feet, left, right, left.
Open out to lines of three.
Repeat dance.

Virginia Reel (America)

Formation:

Longways sets of five couples, facing each other, two yards apart.

Steps:

Skip or walk, slides.

Movements:

Four skips forward, nod to partner.
Four skips backwards.
Four skips forward, do-si-do with partner, passing right shoulders.
Repeat, passing left shoulders.
Four skips forward, right elbow swing with partner.
Repeat, with left elbow swing.
Four skips to meet partner, join hands.
Four slides up the room.
Four slides down the room.
Release hands, four skips back to place.

Single cast. Head couples separate, turn outwards, lead lines down the room, meet partners, join hands, skip up the room.

Double cast. Couples join inside hands, follow head couple down the room.

Head couple forms an arch; other couples skip through the arch back to starting position.

Repeat the dance with a new head couple.

Toast To King Gustav (Sweden)

Formation:

Square sets, boys on the left of the girls, inside hands joined.

Steps:

Walk, skip

Movements:

Head couples walk forward to center, bow or curtsy.
Head couples walk back to place, four steps.
Side couples repeat the above movements.
Head and side couples repeat the above movements.
Side couples raise inside hands to form an arch.
Head couples skip forward to center, release hands, join hands with
    opposite partner, turn and skip through the side arches, release hands,
    return to own partner, and skip round in place.
Head couples form arches, and side couples repeat the above movement.

Square Dance (America)

Formation:

Square sets, boys on the left of the girls.

Steps:

Walk or skip.

Movements:

> *"Square your set."*
(Partners make sure that they are in line, and opposite another
    couple, with backs to the walls.)

> *"Honor your partner and your corner."*
(Partners bow or curtsy to each other, then turn and bow or curtsy to
    their corner.)

> *"Circle left and circle right."*
(All children join hands to form a circle and walk left or right on
    command.)

"All into the center and out again."

(Circle of children walk inwards while raising hands and back out again.)

"Do-si-do your partner; do-si-do your corner."

(Partners face each other, walk forward and pass right shoulders, then back up to place.

Partners turn to face their corners, walk forward and pass left shoulders, then back up to place.)

"Swing your partner; swing your corner."

(Partners face each other, link right elbows and swing around on the spot.

Partners turn to face their corners, link left elbows and swing around on the spot.)

"Promenade your partner."

(Partners stand side by side, with inside hands joined, facing counterclockwise. They walk forward in a circle until back in place.)

"Star right, star left."

(Boys step forward to the center, join right hands, and face clockwise. They walk around in a full circle.

They drop hands, turn around and join left hands, then walk around in a full circle and fall back into place with partner. Repeat with the girls forming the star.)

"Grand right and left."

(Partners face each other, give right hands to each other and pass by. They give left hands to the next person they are facing and pass by. This is repeated all the way around the circle, until partners get back home.)

The above square dance moves are basic to all square dancing. After the children have mastered them, the teacher varies them to avoid monotony. These moves should be taught before commercial square dance records are used, as the latter tend to be too fast for young children to follow.

Ethnic Dances

The Duck Dance (American Indian)

Formation:

Two lines of dancers, hands on hips.

Movements:

As the song begins, leaders for each line move forward, imitating the walk of the duck. They sway first to the right and then to the left, two steps per measure. On the "ho-ke-la-ho," the lines face each other, all dancers make a hand tremelo on their knees, then raise their arms high to indicate flight. At this time the two leaders fly away to the end of the line and the dance continues again with two new leaders. It is important to emphasize that the lines must move together at all times. The proper performance of the dance insured the cooperation of the ducks or other animals during the hunt.

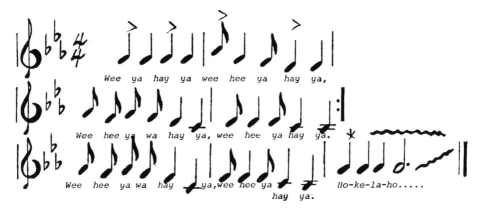

Figure 60. Music for "The Duck Dance." Courtesy of Allyn and Bacon.

Singing Up The Corn (American Indian)

Formation:

One boy stands in the center of the dance area.
Double line of girls at side moves into a single circle.

Movements:

The boy acknowledges the Sun Spirit by facing East. As he slowly turns, his arms move in a wide arc to indicate the passage of the sun from East to West.

In his hands he carries a prayer feather and a small spruce branch.

He now must go and beckon the Corn Maidens to come.

He precedes them by sprinkling a path of corn meal for them to follow.

The Corn Maidens carry small baskets and ears of corn. A drum tremelo signals their entrance.

Entrance is in a double line.

When in the center of the room, the Maidens join in an open circle.

On the first line of the song, the circle moves right.

Step on right foot . . . slide left.

Right . . . slide left.

Sway right, left, right, left.

At the same time keep hands moving from side to side.

Continue this formation throughout the song.

At the end, toss some of the corn into the center of the circle.

The dance may then be repeated to the left.

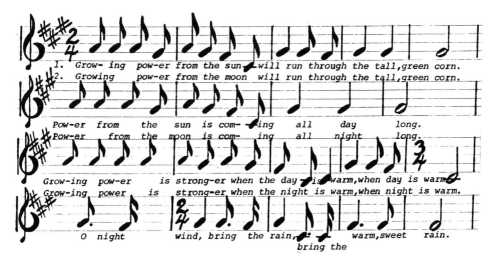

Figure 61. Music for "Singing Up The Corn." Courtesy of Allyn and Bacon.

Dragon Dance (Indonesia)

Formation:

Children stand in Indian file, holding the waist of the child in front of
  them.

Movements:

Children walk in time with the song and as soon as it is finished, the
  "head" of the dragon (the head person in line) chases the "tail." It is
  important not to break the line, so everyone runs. The "tail," of
  course, does his/her best not to get caught, but (s)he may not let go of
  the player in front of him/her. If the tail is caught, (s)he must drop out
  of line and the game starts all over again, with the next-to-last player
  in the line as the new "tail."

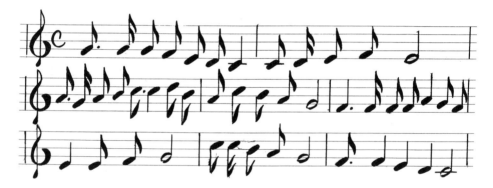

Figure 62. Music for "Dragon Dance." Courtesy of U.S. Committee for UNICEF, and translator
Francine Wicks.

Poi Dance (New Zealand)

Equipment:

Small balls (pois) made from tissue paper inside a plastic bag, with a
  length of string about 18 inches long (see "Improvising Equipment" in
  Chapter X).

Formation:

Lines of children, side by side.

Movements:

Hold one poi in right hand, swing in a circle to right side of body.

Repeat, with right hand in a circle overhead, in front of body.

Repeat with left hand.

With right hand, swing poi in a figure eight across the front of the body.

Repeat with left hand.

Now use the above movements in different combinations.

When the above movements are mastered, use two pois, one in each hand.

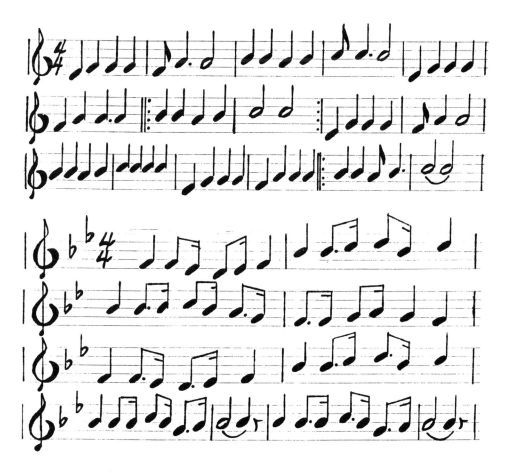

Figure 63. Music for "Poi Dance." World Copyright Control-Viking Sevenseas, P.O. Box 152, Paraparaumu, New Zealand.

Jump Rope Rhymes

Many versions of jump rope rhymes have evolved in different countries. Teachers can use those from their own childhood or the following versions.

Individual:

WORDS	ACTIONS
Jelly in the bowl	Jump rope on spot
Jelly in the bowl	
Wiggy waggy, wiggy waggy	Wiggle hips while jumping
Jelly in the bowl	Jump rope on spot
Teddy bear, teddy bear turn around	Do actions suggested by words
Teddy bear, teddy bear touch the ground	
Teddy bear, teddy bear show your shoe	
Teddy bear, teddy bear that will do	Run out
Grace, Grace dressed in lace	Jump rope on spot
Went upstairs to powder her face	
How many boxes did she use	
One, two, three ...	On "one," do Peppers until tripped
Andy Pandy, sugar and candy	Jump rope on spot
French almond Nuts!	On shouting "Nuts," squat down and twirl rope overhead

With Partner:

House to rent, inquire within	Jump rope on spot
Next door neighbor, please come in	On "in," partner jumps in

In Groups:

Bluebells, cockle shells	Swing rope back and forth
Eevie, ivy, over	On "over," swing it over jumpers' heads
All in together girls	
Never mind the weather girls	Children jump rope,
When I shout your birthday	run out when birth month called
Please jump out	
January, February ... December	
Spanish dancers do the splits	Children jump rope, do actions
Spanish dancers give a high kick	On "Pepper," jump fast

Spanish dancers turn around
Spanish dancers touch the ground
Spanish dancers get out of town
Spanish dancers come back in
Spanish dancers sit on a pin
How many inches did it go in
So pitch, patch, PEPPER
One, two, three . . .

Here comes the teacher   Same as above
With a red hot stick
Wonder what I got in arithmetic
So pitch, patch, PEPPER
One, two, three . . .

I am a girl scout dressed in blue   Children jump rope
These are the actions I can do   On "ease," jump astride
Stand at ease, bend my knees   On "knees," jump to squat
Turn my back on the old tom cat   Turn a full circle

Old Man Daisy   Children jump rope
You're driving me crazy   Move to one end, then the other
Up the ladder, down the ladder   On "T," jump Pepper
One, two, three
Pepper, salt, vinegar,
H. O. T.

Lady, lady at the gate   Children jump rope
Eating cherries from a plate   On "one," jump Pepper
How many cherries did she eat?
One, two, three . . .

Mother, mother I am ill   One child starts jumping.
Send for the doctor to give me   (S)he is joined by others
a pill   as they are named.
In comes the doctor
In comes the nurse
In comes the lady with the
alligator purse

The following verses do not have any specific actions:

Doctor Foster went to Gloucester
In a shower of rain
He stepped in a puddle way up to his middle
And never went there again

Hello, hello, hello, sir
Meet me at the grocer
No, sir
Why sir?
Because I have a cold, sir
Where did you get the cold, sir?
At the North Pole, sir
What were you doing there, sir?
Shooting polar bear, sir
Let me hear you sneeze, sir
Kachoo, kachoo, kachoo, sir

Sally over the water
Sally over the sea
Sally broke a milk bottle
And blamed it on me
Sally told Ma
Ma told Pa
Sally got a scolding
Ha, ha, ha

Have children make up their own fun rhymes to jump rope to.
Teach children to put ropes away neatly.
Fold in half, tie in a knot, hang on the arm of the child gathering up the ropes.

Chapter VI

FITNESS FOR LIFE

Alarm bells have been sounded on the visible increase in obese children and the decline in their physical activity. Their physical inactivity is not off-setting their calorie intake, particularly of fats and sugars: junk food and snacks. This increase in the number of obese children is readily observable at the pre-school and primary grade level. Research indicates that obese young children will become obese adults unless some intervention occurs. That is, increased regular activity and decreased consumption of nonnutritious calories.

In addition to *physical* fitness, today the emphasis is on *health-related* fitness for life.[1]

Physical Fitness Components:

Speed
Strength
Power
Agility
Balance
Endurance

Health-Related Fitness Components:

Muscular strength and endurance (upper body and abdominal)
Aerobic endurance
Flexibility
Body composition

From the very first week of the school year, teachers should be providing activities that cover all the components of health-related fitness along with skill development. It has become increasingly important for

---

[1]Primary grade physical education teachers should consider the fitness education and assessment program *The Prudential FITNESSGRAM* developed by and available from the Cooper Institute for Aerobics Research, 12330 Preston Road, Dallas, Texas 75230.

pre-school and primary physical education teachers to compensate for the inactivity of children by providing daily, vigorous, appropriate activities in which the whole body is involved and the heart rate is raised. Children should be taught to observe changes in their bodies during and after the activity, such as increasing and decreasing pulse rates, breathing rates, body temperatures, and the time it takes to fully recover from vigorous activity. It is equally important that an awareness of "feeling great" be instilled in children at an early age so that involvement in activities becomes a way of life.

A key element in promoting health-related fitness is parental involvement. The process does not stop at the school fence. Parents need to be involved from the beginning of the school year, with a letter informing them about the program plans; the need for their cooperation in providing good nutrition, rest, and activities that will enhance the teacher's efforts in the activity class. Yes, *activity* homework and weekend assignments are essential! Encourage parents to do them with their children. If space is a problem in the home, assign on-the-spot stretch and strengthen routines. Make videos in the activity class for children to check out. This could be a PTA project. Some schools have developed successful parent/child activity nights and Saturdays. A parent/teacher meeting devoted to showcasing the physical education program is a must. Past experience has shown that if a child is performing at a PTA meeting, the chances are that at least one parent will attend.

Teachers must initiate and inform children of the following physiological principles of exercise to improve their fitness levels:

Frequency of Exercise: Daily physical activity is a most desirable goal to set for lifetime patterns.

Time: Thirty minutes of daily activity is recommended.

Intensity: Increasing the *pace* of an activity period is necessary to improve fitness. Gradually increase the *number* of repetitions of exercises; increase the *range* or size of the movements, increase the *speed* of such activities as walking, running, as well as the *distance* covered.

Fitness activities need not be dull or boring. The items in this chapter are traditional physical fitness activities disguised with fun names and approaches.

SHUTTLE FUN RUN

Objective:

To measure agility.

Method:

Two teddy bears (dolls) are placed 5 yards (10 yards) apart.

Teacher times child while (s)he runs from the starting line, beside one teddy, around the other teddy, back to starting line, making 3 (5, etc.) complete trips.

Time is recorded on child's personal chart.

CREEPY FINGERS

Objective:

To practice curl ups.

Method:

Child lies on back on mat, knees bent, hands by side.

Child lifts head and shoulders while sliding hands forward along mat over a taped line.

Teacher records if fingers cross taped line.

Child attempts three times to start.

Then add more attempts.

LONG JUMP BUMP

Objective:

To measure leg power.

Method:

Child does a standing long jump into a pit, along a grassy area, or along a tumbling mat.

Teacher measures distance from starting line to where heels or other body parts land.

Distance is recorded on child's personal chart.

HOT FEET LEAP

Objective:

To measure leg power.

Method:

Child performs a running long jump into a pit or along a tumbling mat.
Teacher measures distance from starting line.
Distance is recorded on child's personal chart.

TARZAN LADDER

Objective:

To measure leg power.

Method:

Teacher draws a "ladder" that increases in width on the ground (see
    Chapter X for "Playground Markings").
Child starts at the narrowest end and runs and leaps across the ladder.
(S)he continues to leap back and forth, up the ladder, until (s)he fails to
    get across.
Teacher records on the child's personal chart how many rungs up the
    ladder the child was successful.

NOSEY PARKER PEEK

Objective:

To measure vertical jumping ability.

Method:

Teacher draws imaginary fences on a wall or on a cardboard chart.
Child stands beside the wall and reaches up and makes a blackboard
    eraser mark.
Child then jumps up and tries to make another eraser mark as high on
    the wall as (s)he can reach.
Teacher measures distance between first and second mark.
Distance is recorded on child's personal chart.

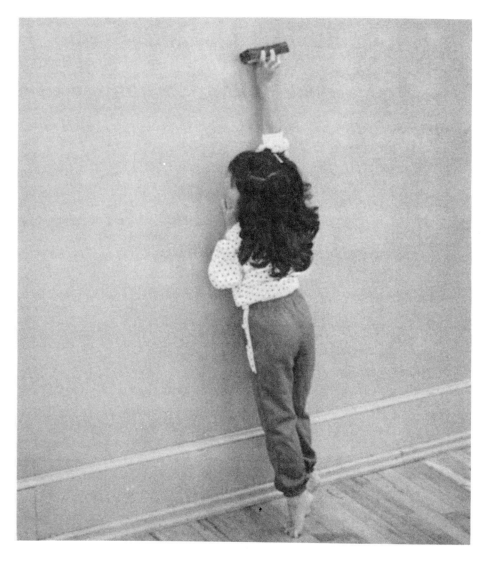

Figure 64. "Reach as high as you can."

FRENCH FRY FLING

Objective:

To measure throwing ability.

Method:

Teacher makes a beanbag shaped like a giant french fry.
Child throws it from starting line as far as possible.
Distance is recorded on child's personal chart.

FITNESS CIRCUIT

Objective:

To increase cardiovascular efficiency, muscular strength and endurance, agility, and balance.

Method:

Place markers at corners of activity area.
Use old juice cartons or bleach bottles filled with sand to keep them upright.
Decorate them as characters, such as Teddy, Mickey Mouse, Pocahontas, Batman, Space Man, Barney (see "Improvising Equipment" in Chapter X).
For a fun run, ask the children to line up beside Teddy and run to visit Mickey Mouse, Batman, etc.
Increase the distance gradually.
Designate activities to be done at each station.

STATIONS	ACTIVITY EXAMPLES
Teddy	3 frog jumps around him
Barney	balance walk along rope
Batman	beanbag toss for distance (or accuracy)
Pocahontas	3 bunny jumps around her
Space Man	practice rope jumping, count how many
Mickey Mouse	"Nosey Parker Peek"

PROGRESS CHARTS

Wall Charts:

Use large cardboard sheets.
Record the children's names at the side.
Record the activity along the top.
Record times, distances, or successful completion of an activity.
Use stars to indicate best performance of each child.

Sample of Progress Chart

LOOK WHAT I CAN DO!									
My name is	Long Jump Bump			French Fry Fling			Nosey Parker Peek	Tarzan Ladder	Shuttle Fun Run
1. Sally	3	3 ½	4	10	12	12*			
2. John	3 ½	3 ½	4 ½	11	12	14*			
3. Michael	2	2 ¾	3	9	9	11*			
4. Maria	2 ½	3	3 ½	6	7*	6			
5. James	4	4	2 ½						
6. Gina									

*Best effort

POSITIVE PROGRESS REPORT FOR PARENTS

Use butcher paper to make large books for the children to use as report cards to take home and keep. (It has been observed that they read them constantly.)

Teacher or child writes on one page what they can do and illustrates the activity.

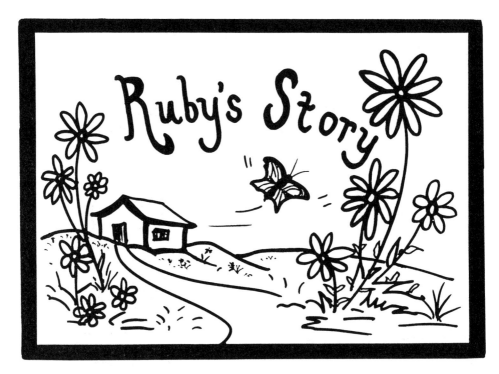

Figure 65. Report Card Cover.

I can

roll like a

jump like a

jump like a

shake like a

fly like a

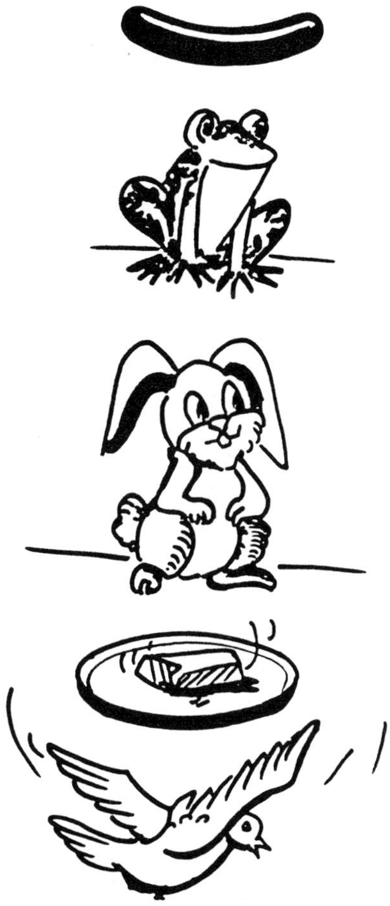

Figure 66. Sample Report Card Page.

I can dance
like a ballerina.

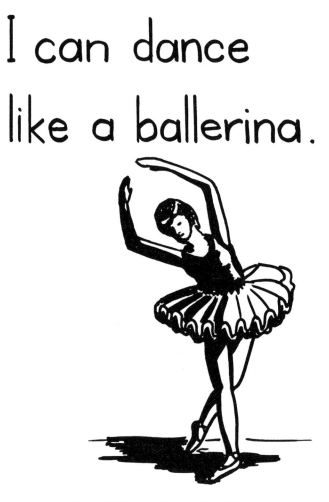

Figure 67. Sample Report Card Page.

---

[2]Primary teachers should consider rope jumping as a fitness activity. The Jump Rope for Heart program is a worthwhile endeavor. For further information, write Jump Rope for Heart Program, American Alliance for Health, Physical Education, Recreation and Dance, 1900 Association Drive, Reston VA 22091.

Chapter VII

WATER CONFIDENCE PLAY

This chapter is directed at those teachers who are fortunate enough to have access to a *shallow* pool. Few public schools have pools, so most of the following activities shall be conducted in YWCA and YMCA facilities, private pools and clubs, and city pools.

The pool water level should not exceed the waist level of the children, and there should be a rail or ledge for the children to grasp.

Safety factors must be stressed:

There must be adequate adult supervision at all times and a low pupil/teacher ratio.

No child should be in the water alone.

Each child should have a partner to look after during the lesson.

High standards of hygiene should be stressed:

Pools and surroundings must be clean and properly maintained.

Children with recent or current infections should not participate.

Children must go to the toilet before the lesson.

Children should shower and use a footbath before entering the pool.

The aim of water confidence play is to involve the children in enjoyable water activities so that they will feel comfortable and at ease in water. Water play is a necessary prelude to learning to float and to swim. It is at this stage that the children learn to breathe easily, to submerge, to open their eyes underwater, and to propel themselves through the water. Most importantly, they should be relaxing and having fun.

The following activities are divided into three sections:

Getting into the water.

Going under the water.

Moving through the water.

GETTING INTO THE WATER

Humpty Dumpty:

Child sits on edge of pool; on "fall," child slides into water.

Making Waves:

Child faces side of pool, holds on to rail, and moves body forward and back.

Follow the Leader:

Child walks across pool, hands on waist of child in front, and bounces up and down.

Bouncing Ball:

Child jumps up and down in the water.

Washing Machine:

Child places hands on hips and twists from side to side.

Speedboats:

Child moves around pool, with arms stretched back, and mouth at water level blowing out to make engine sound.

Whirlpool:

Child holds arms out wide and turns around slowly to stir up water.

Elephants Bathing:

Child cups hands and pours water over head.

Birds Bathing:

Child bends knees, folds arms across body (wings), flaps wings up, jumps up, and repeats, making lots of splash.

Here, There, Where:

Children run where teacher points; on "where," they jump up and down on the spot.

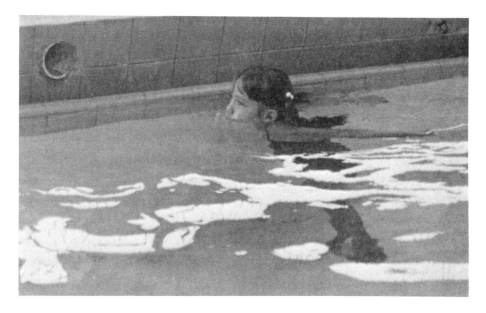

Figure 68. Speedboats.

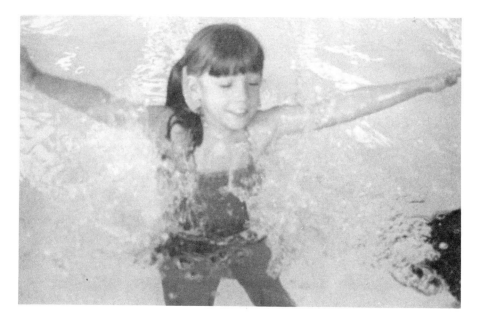

Figure 69. Birds Bathing.

Seaplanes:

Child walks around pool with arms stretched wide; lands with a splash.

Crocodiles:

Children walk across pool in lines of three; leader zigzags to make tail waggle.

Balls:

Child plays with large rubber ball; pushes ball with hands, head, elbow; hugs ball; tries to lie on it.

GETTING UNDER THE WATER

Train Thru the Tunnel:

Children play "Follow The Leader." Teacher holds a kickboard at edge of pool for children to go under; encourages them to sound whistles and to open eyes while underwater.

Circus Dog:

Child stands on edge of pool, jumps into plastic hoop, submerges, and goes under edge of hoop.

Polar Bear:

Child stands in water beside hoop, submerges and comes up through hole in ice (hoop).

Frogs Catching Flies:

Child submerges until only eyes are above water, jumps up, reaches up with one hand (tongue) and pretends to catch a fly, and resubmerges.

Seesaws:

With partners, hands joined, one child submerges while other child comes up.

Pop Goes the Weasel:

In groups; on "pop," children submerge.

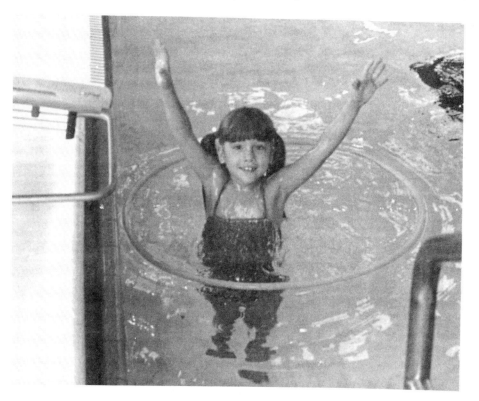

Figure 70. Polar Bear.

Jack in the Box:

Children bounce up and down while they say: "Jack in the box jumps up, Jack in the box jumps down!" On "down," children submerge.

Big A:

"Big A, little a, Bouncing B
Cat's in the Cupboard and Can't See Me!"
Children jump up and down; on "me," children submerge their faces so teacher can't see them.

I Clap:

*"I clap up high . . .
I clap down low . . .
I jump, jump, jump . . .
And down I go! . . . "*

Children do actions of verse.

Submarines:

Child walks around under the water with hand (periscope) up, comes up
   for a breath, and goes down again.

Turtles:

Child hugs knees, *takes a big breath,* and tries to float.

MOVING THROUGH THE WATER[1]

Floating Bodies:

Child stands with back to rail, reaches back over shoulders to grasp rail,
   takes a big breath, and lets legs float to surface.
Child faces rail, lightly grasps it with fingertips, takes a big breath, puts
   face in water, lets legs float up, and drifts away from the rail.

Towing Logs:

With partner, one child cups hands under back of head and neck of other
   child who floats on back, breathing relaxed, gently moving legs and
   arms, moving around the pool.
With partner, one behind the other, front child walks forward, back child
   holds front child's hands and floats face down, gently moving legs,
   inhaling, exhaling while face is submerged.
Repeat above movements using a foam kickboard instead of a partner.

Gliding:

Child stands back from edge of pool in front lunge position, arms
   extended forward at shoulder height; pushes off with feet, inhales,
   submerges face and glides towards rail, breathing out underwater.

Sculling:

Child lies back in water, breathes in, gently swings long legs up and
   down, sculls (wiggles) hands at sides.
When the children have mastered the above progressions, they are ready
   to learn the traditional swimming strokes.

---

[1]For additional activities, consult: YMCA (1987). *Y Skippers, An Aquatic Program for Children Five and
Under.* Champaign, IL: Human Kinetics.
Langendorfer, S. and Bruya, L. (1995). *Aquatic Readiness.* Champaign, IL: Human Kinetics.

Chapter VIII

PHYSICAL EDUCATION
FOR SPECIAL POPULATIONS

PHYSICAL EDUCATION FOR THE DISABLED

In 1975, the Education for All Handicapped Children's Act, Public Law 94-142, was signed into law. The 1990 Individuals with Disabilities Education Act reinforced this law, ensuring that all children will be included, not excluded from education. It is based on the assumption that all disabled children are capable of benefiting from a free, appropriate, public education and related services. The law requires that these children be educated in the least restrictive environment, must have an Individualized Education Program, must have access to their records, and have due process in their placement and program.

The disabled served under PL 94-142 are categorized as follows:

1. Mentally retarded
2. Emotionally disturbed
3. Learning disabled
4. Orthopedically handicapped
5. Visually handicapped
6. Hearing impaired
7. Speech communication impaired
8. Other health impairments

Physical education is a requirement under the law, and recreation is a component of related services. These services must be prescribed in the Individualized Education Program for each disabled child.

Recognizing that disabled children are more alike than different from the nondisabled, every effort should be made to mainstream them into regular classes. The physical education class is often the first and most appropriate place to begin the mainstreaming process.

Unfortunately, to comply with PL 94-142, disabled children have been mainstreamed into already overcrowded physical education classes with little chance of these children receiving the individualized attention and help needed for skill development and improvement. In this situation, it is suggested that the highly skilled children in the class tutor the disabled children one-on-one for *short* segments of the class period, but not to the detriment of their own skill improvement and enjoyment. Parent volunteers and aides should also be enlisted to assist the disabled children.

Care must be taken to see that disabled children are not subject to ridicule or harassment when mainstreamed. These children may have already experienced failure in the classroom, and need to experience success, no matter how small, in physical education. Here, they can increase their self-esteem, can socialize, and be accepted by the nondisabled. Mainstreaming is a two-way street, and the nondisabled children can also benefit. They can become more accepting of those who are different if the physical education teacher creates a positive atmosphere.

The physical education teacher must insist on a full disclosure of the children's disabilities, physicians' reports on any limitations on participation, and clearances to participate. Too often in the past children's disabling conditions have not been disclosed to the teacher on the grounds that attaching labels to children would result in treating them differently. In many cases, these children with disabilities *need* different or individualized help, determined by a knowledge and understanding of their conditions.

If disabled children are not able to benefit from mainstreaming in regular activity classes, then adapted activity classes must be provided, *keeping the teacher/child ratio low.*

Whether mainstreamed or in special activity classes, adaptations will have to be made to the disabling condition of the child. General modifications for the less able include:

Simplifying the rules of a game.

Using smaller, softer balls.

Lowering the basketball goals.

Decreasing the size of a team.

Enlarging goals or target areas.

Slowing down music for dances.

Giving children more time to master skills.

Following are suggestions for adaptations for specific disabilities:

Mentally Retarded

These children's motor skill development parallels normal children's but proceeds at a slower rate.

Posture and body mechanics are poor.

Their learning rate is very slow.

They must learn and relearn.

They need one-to-one direct teaching with short, simple instructions.

They need to be manipulated through a movement from the rear to avoid confusion in direction.

They need large muscle activities and the opportunity to release tension through body movement.

They need to develop lifetime recreational skills such as dance, swimming, track and field.

Preparation for the Special Olympics can be a viable program in itself.

They need to improve their total body fitness.

Most important of all, they need a teacher with patience and sensitivity who will be pleased with even the smallest improvement in performance.

Emotionally Disturbed

These children may have accompanying behavioral problems.

They *may* be defiant, hostile, frustrated, unpredictable, withdrawn, defensive, stubborn, unwilling to participate.

They can benefit from vigorous activity to release tensions and frustrations.

They may need a great deal of individual attention just to get them to conform to the rules and procedures of the class.

Learning Disabled

These children have probably already experienced failure in the classroom.

They are often clumsy and have poorly developed gross motor skills.

They need to experience success, no matter how small, in the activity class.

They need simple, achievable goals.

They need encouragement and praise for what they do well.

Do not allow them to be harassed by other children for dropping a ball, missing a basket, running the wrong way.

Do not allow children to choose teams and have the learning disabled chosen last.

Orthopedically Handicapped

These children may be confined to wheel chairs, on crutches, or in limb braces.

Their physical therapist must furnish a report to include their physical condition: muscle tone, range of motion, posture and movement capacity, and limitations and recommendations for physical education.

These children are capable of participating in many activities with adaptations.

They need a health-related fitness program.

They need to develop lifetime recreational skills.

Successful programs have been developed in:

Wheelchair basketball.

Wheelchair square dance.

Bowling.

Swimming.

Rhythmic activities—manipulating hoops, streamers, pois.

Visually Handicapped

These children need activities which pair them with sighted children.

They need clear signals such as a whistle, or bell, to signify "STOP" and listen for directions.

Successful programs have been developed in:

Beep ball—modified softball with a beeper in the ball.

Roller skating.

Folk dance.

Swimming—with roped lanes.

Hearing Impaired

These children can participate in all physical education activities.

Caution must be exercised in climbing activities, as there may be a balance impairment.

The teacher needs to remember to face the child directly when giving instructions.

The teacher should, if possible, remove excessive background noises.

The teacher should learn sign language necessary to referee games, and to indicate directions, infringements, etc.

Flags raised or lowered and large arm signals will help the children.

Speech Communication Impaired

These children can participate in all physical education activities.

They need to be protected from harassment by insensitive children.

The teacher needs to be patient while they try to express themselves.

They need to develop *lifetime* recreational skills to enable them to socialize outside the school environment.

Health Impaired

This category includes those who suffer from respiratory disorders, cardiac disorders, diabetes, allergies, epilepsy, kidney disease, cancer, hemophilia, etc.

They are often more in need of physical activity than the normal child, but are often totally excluded because of their health.

A physician's report must be furnished with a full disclosure of their condition, their limitations, and recommendations for physical activity.

These children must be carefully observed and monitored during the activity.

A knowledge of emergency action and CPR is a must for their teacher.

Seriously Obese

These children are considered disabled, as their condition interferes with normal day-to-day life.

They need private, individualized assessment, counseling, and goal-setting.

They need a physician's report and recommendations for their individualized exercise and activity program.

They need nutrition education and an immediate change in diet.

They need encouragement, and a genuine attitude of concern on the part of the teacher.

They need to be protected from harassment by insensitive children.

The 1988 AAHPERD *PHYSICAL BEST* health-related fitness program and assessment is ideal for disabled children, because it contains participation and personal goals awards achievable by them.[1]

Because the activities in this book are arranged from *simple* to *complex*, they lend themselves to adaptation for the disabled. As each challenge is accomplished, the teacher moves the child to the next one. No complex activities should be attempted unless the child has exhibited *success* and *strength* in the simpler activities.

CROSSING THE LANGUAGE BRIDGE
IN PHYSICAL EDUCATION

Limited English Proficient (LEP) children increase in number annually in the pre-school and primary grades. Sometimes an activity class will contain several immigrant children from different countries and/or non-English speaking families. The activity class is an ideal place to help the LEP children cross the language bridge. Through a bombardment of their senses, the children can:

Hear (the challenge).

See (the action or reaction of other children).

Do (the action themselves).

Say (the action words).

There are two main methods of presenting activity materials to children:

1. **Show:** The traditional method, where the teacher or another child shows the children what to do and how to do it. Clearly this would be the most appropriate and effective method to use with LEP children to start with.

2. **Sow:** The movement education approach, where the teacher sows the seed of an idea, in the children's minds, through verbalization for them to develop and respond with a physical action. This method could be used as the children's grasp of English strengthens.

Teachers must be very sensitive to the culture shock some immigrant children are experiencing. Common, everyday habits in one country, such as wearing shorts for activity, may be a traumatic experience for

---

[1]For more details of the *PHYSICAL BEST* program, write American Alliance for Health, Physical Education, Recreation and Dance, 1900 Association Drive, Reston, VA 22901.

new immigrants. Teachers should make allowances for such children during the enculturation period.

Bilingual Education and Physical Education

Bilingual education has been defined as instruction in two languages; in some or all school subjects. Its purpose is to enhance the children's chances of academic success through the use of the language they bring to school from their homes. Some proponents of bilingual education in America have as their goals the transition from the native language to fluency in English, in order that children may function and succeed in a predominantly English-speaking country. Other educators have as their goals the maintenance of truly bilingual children, fluent and functional in both their own cultures and in an English-speaking society. This can be accomplished either gradually or by immersion in English.

If there is a large number of Hispanic children in a school, the following methods can be used in an activity class to give the children sound movement experiences and help them cross the language bridge from Spanish to English or from English to Spanish. The material is directed at four different groups of children:

1. A class of Spanish language dominant children.
2. A class with a mixture of Spanish dominant and English dominant children.
3. A class of bilingual children who are relatively balanced in the use of English and Spanish.
4. A class of English dominant children with a few Spanish dominant children.

How to Present the Material:

The composition of the class will dictate how the materials will be used. For example:

1. *Spanish dominant class.* In this situation, the teacher should initially present the challenges in Spanish and gradually introduce them in English.
2. *Mixture of Spanish dominant and English dominant class.* Depending on the numbers involved, the teacher should present the challenges in English and reinforce them in Spanish for those who do not understand at first. In this situation, not only will the Spanish

dominant children *hear* the challenges in English, but they will also *see* how the English dominant children react. In addition, the English dominant children will hear the movement challenges in Spanish and in the process will become familiar with a second language.

3. *Bilingual class.* The challenges should be given in English but reinforced in Spanish if it appears that some children do not understand. This exposes the children to the challenge in two languages: they can see how other children are responding with movement and they can do the action themselves.

4. *English dominant class with a few Spanish dominant or bilingual children.* The challenges should be given in English but reinforced in Spanish for the minority group.

Basic Challenges Vocabulary:

ENGLISH	SPANISH
Can you . . . ?	¿Pueden . . . ?
Let me see you . . .	Déjenme verlos . . .
Show me how you can . . .	Enseñenme como . . .
Try to . . .	Traten de . . .

How to Build Up a Challenge:

Basic Movement: Run	Corran
Basic Movement with one variation:	
Can you run slowly?	¿Pueden correr despacio? (lento)
Basic Movement with two variations:	
Can you run slowly in a circle?	¿Pueden correr despacio en un círculo?

Other Ways That the Two Languages Can Be Used in Physical Education:

1. Record scores of games in two languages.
2. Label equipment and equipment boxes.
3. Record long and high jump results.
4. Record heights and weights of children.
5. Write class instructions on the blackboard.
6. Write action words on the blackboard.
7. Conduct a lesson with all challenges in English, and all praises in Spanish. Reverse this in another lesson.
8. Count for jumps, etc. in English or Spanish.

9. Teach Hispanic folk dances and singing games; translate the words, discuss the cultural heritage.
10. Place a large silhouette of a body on the gym wall. Label the body parts in both English and Spanish.
11. Pair Limited English Proficient children with English dominant children.

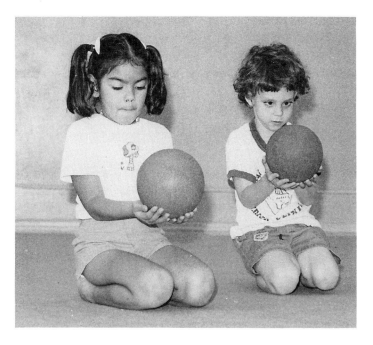

Figure 71. Pair Limited English Proficient children with English dominant children.

PHYSICAL EDUCATION FOR
THE GIFTED AND TALENTED

Gifted and talented children have been categorized as follows:

1. *Academic ability:* Those who exhibit high intellectual potential.
2. *Creative ability:* Those who exhibit creative thinking and creativity in the visual and performing arts.
3. *Psychosocial ability:* Those who exhibit outstanding leadership qualities.
4. *Kinesthetic ability:* Those who exhibit superior psychomotor ability.

The needs of the gifted and talented children are similar to their classmates but may differ in *degree, quality,* and *fulfillment.* Their physical education program must dovetail into their total education program's goals. That is:

1. To provide opportunities to reach their highest potential.
2. To provide opportunities to think creatively and to seek original solutions to challenges.
3. To provide opportunities to develop positive self-concepts.
4. To provide opportunities to interact with children of similar abilities and to develop a sensitivity to their needs.
5. To provide opportunities to interact with children with lesser abilities in order to operate with ease in the "real" world.

The physical education class is an ideal setting for achieving the above goals. The activities included in this book provide a wealth of opportunities for the gifted and talented child to use a flexible approach to problem solving and to create imaginative solutions. Particularly in responding to challenges, the individual child has a rare opportunity to exhibit his/her creativity and unique responses. For example, in "Similes," when the teacher asks the class to "wiggle like a bug that has just been sprayed" or to "fly like a bird that has eaten too much," the creative child's imagination can really take wings. Often, in creative dance, the imaginative child, in a heterogeneous group, emerges as the leader to impose his/her patterns on the others. When a class is asked to show the teacher five different ways to bounce a ball, the imaginative child is quick to accomplish this. In gymnastics, when the class is asked to combine their vocabulary of "rolls" into a "movement sentence," the creatively thinking child responds uniquely.

In response to the efforts of the gifted and talented child, the physical education teacher must be enthusiastic, must praise, and must give the child his/her moment of glory by asking the other children to observe and/or to copy the unique response to the challenge. This can enhance the self-esteem of the creative child and can inspire other children to seek different responses to the challenges.

Chapter IX

METHODS OF TEACHING PHYSICAL EDUCATION

This chapter is directed mainly to teacher educators. However, parents, latch-key program directors, day care directors, and others responsible for planning activity programs for young children can use the materials presented here to their advantage in developing lessons and developmental programs. Teacher aides will enhance their value to teachers by becoming familiar with the contents of this chapter.

Student teachers will do well to study the materials presented in order to gain confidence during their practicums.

PLANNING A PHYSICAL EDUCATION PROGRAM

The planning of a program is contingent upon the following factors:
Climate

Facilities and surfaces

Equipment

Size of the class

Imagination of the teacher

Climate:

A cold and/or wet day dictates vigorous activities. Children should not stand around waiting for turns. Walking activities, such as in "Singing Games," should be done skipping or running. Hops and jumps, interspersed with stretching activities, will make for a vigorous lesson. Maximum activity in the alloted time should be the goal.

On a hot, dry, or humid day, the pace of the lesson should be slowed down. Use more stretching activities. Introduce new activities, such as tumbling, with children demonstrating. Make sure children have access to drinking water.

Always have a contingency plan for inclement days. Do not wait until the bad weather arrives. The following activities are suggested for bad weather days in a confined space:

Finger plays

Verses

Singing games

Line dances

Reel dances

Square dance moves—demonstrated and walked through

Table games

Films

Guest speaker

Health education topics: fitness, pulse taking, relaxation techniques, fat cells growth

Facilities and Surfaces:

Most pre-school and primary grade activity takes place outside on blacktop, grass, or dirt. Teachers who are outside for all lessons must choose from the activities in this book which lend themselves to the outdoors. They will, by necessity, be restricted in activities involving lying, rolling, sitting, etc. However, they should look for possible indoor areas such as cafetoriums, stages, hallways, breezeways and surplus class-rooms that could be converted into activity rooms. A few lucky teachers have access to an indoor wooden floor or carpet area. These teachers will be able to make full use of the activities in this book.

The surfaces available will dictate the footwear used. Ideally, young children should exercise in bare feet; so, when a smooth floor or carpet is available, they should be encouraged to take off their footwear. Outdoors, on hard or rough surfaces, the children should be encouraged to wear lightweight sports shoes rather than heavy cowboy boots or street shoes.

Hard playground surfaces should have plenty of markings, to be used either in the activity period or at recess. If the same area is used by the upper grades, different-colored paint should be used to distinguish the primary grade markings (see Chapter X, "Playground Markings").

Equipment:

Most teachers will have to make do with a minimum supply of equipment provided by school systems. There may be in the playground a few horizontal bars, a ladder, and a jungle gym. All of these can be utilized for small-group activities, while the other children use balls, beanbags, hoops, etc. No program should be restricted through lack of equipment. Many commercial items can be made by the teacher, the children, parents, or the school district physical plant workers. The golden rule is never to buy what can be improvised (see "Improvising Equipment" in Chapter X).

Size of the Class:

Although pre-school activity class sizes have low caregiver/child ratios, often with aides to help, kindergarten and primary grade physical education classes continue to be overcrowded with much too high teacher/children ratios. This results in reduced opportunities for individualized attention in skill development and practice at a stage when young children need that attention. Additionally, overcrowding children who are moving and using playground equipment increases the chances of accidents occurring. Activity classes should be no larger than regular academic classes.

Imagination of the Teacher:

This is the most critical factor in the planning and development of an activity program. For here the possibilities are limitless, and the program is only as narrow or as broad as the teacher's imagination. There may be restrictions in the line of climate, class size, facilities, surfaces and equipment, but an imaginative teacher will not allow these to impede his/her program. The activities in this book should be utilized to their fullest extent and should then become a springboard for more ideas from the imaginative teacher.

PROGRAM PIES

An activity program can be likened to a pie with various activities making up the segments. In the past, segments of the pie have been unbalanced. Depending on the background or lack of confidence of the teacher, large segments were filled with free play or calisthenics and small segments contained dance and beginning tumbling.

The following are unacceptable program pies:

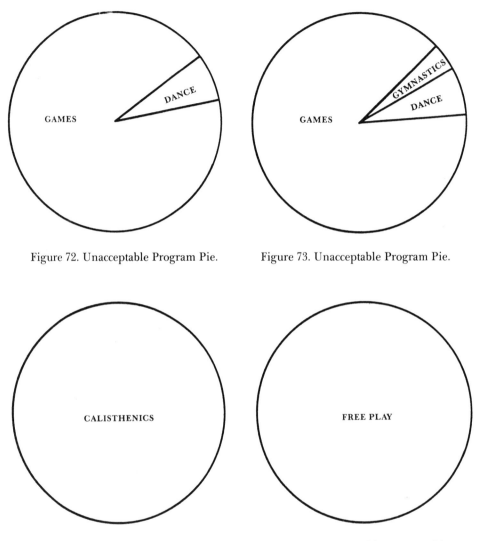

Figure 72. Unacceptable Program Pie.   Figure 73. Unacceptable Program Pie.

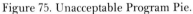

Figure 74. Unacceptable Program Pie.   Figure 75. Unacceptable Program Pie.

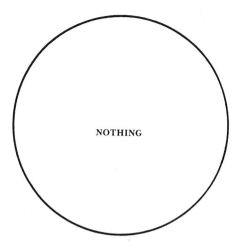

Figure 76. Unacceptable Program Pie.

An "ideal" program pie would look like this:

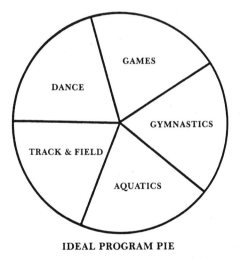

IDEAL PROGRAM PIE

Figure 77. Ideal Program Pie.

A "realistic" program pie would look like this:

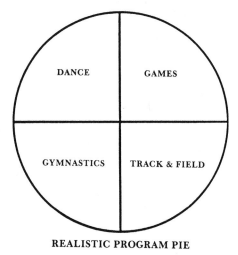

REALISTIC PROGRAM PIE

Figure 78. Realistic Program Pie.

LESSON PLANS

All primary activity lessons should be structured. This is in contrast to pre-school "free play" periods or recess.

A simple lesson should have a beginning, a middle, and an end. It should be psychologically as well as physiologically stimulating. There should be a rhythm of "Puff! Stretch! and Strengthen" throughout the lesson.

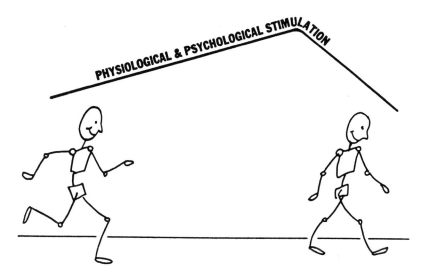

Figure 79. A lesson should be physiologically and psychologically stimulating.

A traditional lesson is structured as follows:

Warm up—teacher directed

Stretch and strengthen exercises

Skill teach

Skill practice

Skill apply in a game, dance, or gymnastics station

Quietening activity

Evaluation

A movement education lesson is structured as follows:

Free activity for early arrivals

Vigorous activity—whole body movements—teacher directed

Specific skill practice

Specific skill refine

Skill use in a game, dance, or gymnastic station

Quietening activity

Evaluation

Twenty-minute to thirty-minute lessons daily are appropriate for preschool and primary grades.

During a lesson there should be a progression whereby the children work on their own, then in pairs, then in small groups, and finally in teams. The lesson must be challenging and fun. It must contain something for everyone, particularly the lesser skilled. Some busy noise is permitted but chaotic noise is not.

METHODS

"Show" Method

In the "show" or traditional method of teaching physical education, the teacher shows the children what to do and they copy or, the teacher has a child demonstrate. Limitations of this method are:

The teacher does most of the work. (S)he poses the problem and provides the answer.

The children are only involved in imitating the teacher's actions.

The teacher will tend to teach only that which (s)he can do or feels confident to demonstrate.

There is a tendency to expect a uniform action from all the children regardless of size, shape, or ability. Therefore, there are always going to be some children who experience failure.

There is very little scope for individual interpretation or variation of movement.

The class tends to move at a set level regardless of a range of ability within the class.

"Sow" Method

In the "sow" method, the teacher sows the seed of an idea in the children's minds through verbalization for the children to develop and respond with a physical action. This method is commonly referred to as the "movement education" approach to teaching physical education.

Characteristics of the "sow" method are:

Emphasis is placed on the efficient use of the whole body.

The teacher provides challenges that will exploit and extend the children physically and mentally so that they must *think before they move, while they move,* and *after they have moved.*

The teacher need not be a performer or an athlete but should become a skilled *verbalizer* who can draw *original* movements from children.

(S)he does this, not by demonstrating actions, nor by leading the class in exercises, but by throwing out verbal challenges which the children are required to respond to with an *action* of their own.

The teacher poses challenges such as:

> *"Can you . . . "*
> *"Let me see you . . . "*
> *"Show me how you can . . . "*
> *"Try to . . . "*

The children are allowed to find their own personal space in the designated general space, rather than be assigned to lines, circles, and squares.

The activities are not done to cadence but are performed at the children's own speed. This allows individuals to jump higher and longer, to stretch further, to finish earlier or later.

Maximum use is made of the activity time, with a minimum of standing around waiting for a turn.

Traditional equipment and improvised equipment is used in a nontraditional manner. For example, balls are balanced on tummies or carried between the feet.

At first, young children who are not familiar with this method will tend to wait for their teacher or their classmates to show them how to "wobble like Jell-O™ on a plate" or to "flap like a flag on a windy day." At this point, the teacher should praise the child who is interpreting a verbal challenge in a different way, so that other children may get the idea that an original action is most desirable. However, all efforts, copied or otherwise, *that basically fulfill the challenge* should be praised so that the children experience positive reinforcement for their efforts.

BASIC MOVEMENTS

Basic movements form the foundation on which all whole body movements are developed. They can be divided as follows:

LOCOMOTOR MOVEMENTS (Movements which take you from place to place)	NON–LOCOMOTOR MOVEMENTS (Movements done on the spot)
Walk	Bend
Run	Stretch
Jump	Twist
Leap	
Hop	

In the activity program, we are concerned with giving children many different experiences in these movements to increase their all-round efficiency and quality of movement. We start with the very simple movements and proceed to the more complex when the simple have been mastered. For example, there is no point in trying to teach children a complicated folk dance, involving such steps as Pas de Basques and Polkas, when they are unable to walk or skip with ease. Neither is there any point in trying to teach children a lay-up shot in basketball when they cannot run and dribble a ball well.

In the five traditional areas of an activity program, the basic movements reappear. They are varied or adapted according to the type of activity involved.

Games and Sports:

Basic movements are adapted to a bat, a ball, a playing area, a set of rules, a teammate, an opponent.

Gymnastics:

Basic movements are adapted to a floor area, a piece of small apparatus, a piece of large apparatus, a partner, a group.

Track and Field:

Basic movements are adapted to a running lane, a set distance, a clock, a pit, a ball (throwing), a teammate, an opponent, a hurdle.

Dance:

Basic movements are combined into dance steps and used to create dance patterns; are adapted to a specific rhythm, feeling, idea (alone, with a partner, in a traditional dance or singing game); or to a piece of small apparatus (ball, hoop, beanbag, etc.); or to instruments (piano, percussion).

Aquatics:

Basic movements are adapted to the medium of water.

How Do We Vary the Basic Movements?

An activity program would be very dull if all it contained were the basic movements. Therefore, the teacher must introduce variations of these movements so that the children are fully extended. Each week, a teacher should examine his/her program to see that a majority of the variations listed here have been experienced by the children.

Variations:

1. Direction: Forward, backwards, sideways, diagonal, patterns

   Examples: *"Walk around the room in your very own circle...*
   Jump around the room and make a banana shape on the floor...
   Make any animal shape on the floor as you run..."

2. Level: High, medium, low

   Examples: *"Walk like a little man...*
   Leap high to touch the stars...
   Stretch up like a giraffe...
   Crawl under a very low fence..."

3. Force: Light, medium, heavy

   Examples: *"Run towards me like a very light elf...*
   Walk away from me stamping your feet like a giant..."

4. Speed: Slow, medium, fast, accelerate, decelerate, even rhythm, uneven rhythm

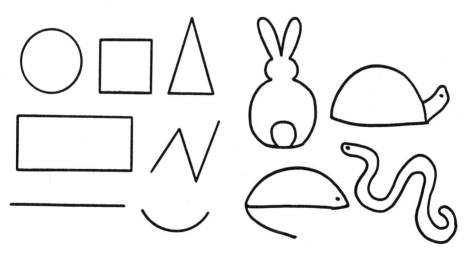

Figure 80. Geometrical patterns.   Figure 81. Animals.

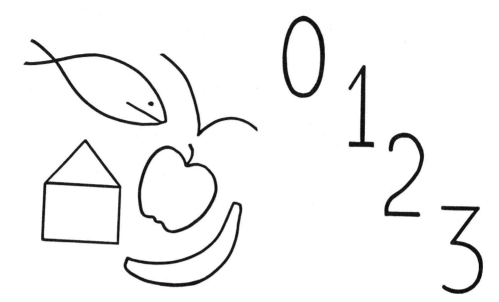

Figure 82. Objects.   Figure 83. Numbers.

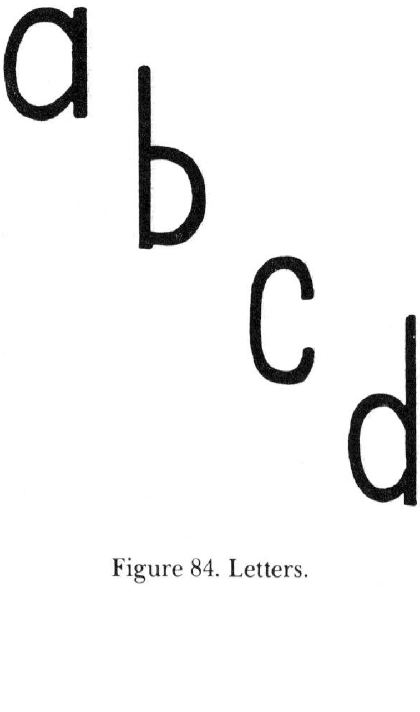

Figure 84. Letters.

Examples: *"Listen to my drum. When it beats slowly, run slowly.*
When it beats fast, run very fast...
Follow the leader, skipping... now galloping...
now sliding... now walking... "

5. Space: Large, medium, small; wide, narrow

Examples: *"Walk with very small steps... now with big giant steps...*
Let me see you take big jumps towards me and little jumps backwards...
Make yourself as fat as a cat... as thin as a pin... "

6. Emotion: Frightened, happy, sad, curious, proud, tired, excited, etc.; characters, animals

Examples:
In this box I have something strange. Come around me and peek inside.
You are very curious...
Now you are frightened and run away... "

CORRELATING PHYSICAL EDUCATION WITH OTHER SUBJECTS

Many of the activities in this book correlate with learning in the classroom. For example, when changing direction, the children are asked to move in different geometrical shapes such as circles, squares, and triangles. In the process of moving and thinking, they are learning about these shapes, which they will encounter in mathematics. They see the shape and make the shape as they walk, run, jump, etc.

When using stretch ropes, the children are also making and learning to recognize shapes: geometrical, flowers, animals, etc. In this same activity, the children are being made aware of the concepts of size: large, small, wide, narrow, big, little, as they manipulate their ropes.

In many activities, the children are learning the ordinal numbers as they are instructed to go first, second, third, etc., in line. In group work, they will learn firsthand how many children are needed to make pairs, groups of three, four, or more.

In prepositional challenges, using boxes or hoops, the children are learning unconsciously that a preposition indicates direction. They hear the preposition and move in the direction indicated. For example: run *around* your hoop, jump *across* your hoop, hop *into* your box. In these same prepositional challenges, the children hear action words (verbs), such as jump, run, hop, and leap, and then do the action.

In beanbag and ball activities, the children are developing spatial awareness as they move in space and become aware of other children's needs for personal space. They are making distance judgements when tossing beanbags or balls through either a hoop or a window made with a stretch rope; when throwing or rolling a ball at a target box, when throwing and catching alone, or with a friend; and when kicking a ball for accuracy or distance. An imaginative teacher will have the children measure the distances that they have thrown or kicked the ball.

In "Similes," not only are the children developing their imaginations, but they are also being exposed to comparisons and action words. For example: *"Wiggle like a bug that has just been sprayed."*

In all activities, it is hoped that the children's imaginations will be exercised, but in particular the sections on "Similes," "Hats" and "Creative Dance" should promote imaginative action. In the latter activity, the children should be encouraged, with the teacher's help, to write up their original dances in a large butcher paper book, to name the dances, and to draw the kinds of costumes they would like the dancers to wear when doing their dances. This is an excellent opportunity for correlations with language arts and fine arts.

TEACHING HINTS

General:

Be prepared.
Know the material.
Have equipment ready.
Learn the children's names. Use tags if necessary.
Have some activity to keep the children busy if they must wait in line.
Cut off an activity when it drags.
Move around the area, observing all the children.
If working with one group, see that the other children are busy with hoops, beanbags, etc.

Organization:

Set boundaries for the class and insist that the children keep inside.
Have the children walk around the area.
Have a "listening line," or place, for the children to assemble for instructions, demonstrations, etc.
Bring the children in close for instructions, then spread out.
Have them sit, squat, or kneel so they can see and be seen.
Use playground markings: circles, lines, etc.

Ask the children to put their toes on the edge of these lines.
Do not have the children facing into the sun.

Spacing:

Ask the children to find their very own space.
Ask them to stretch their arms sideways, then twirl them forward and backwards, without touching anyone.
Encourage the children to move in their own space and not to enter anyone else's space.

Moving:

Station-to-station movement can get confusing if not organized.
Use "Follow the Leader," with basic movements to start, and then with animal moves such as bunny jumps, spider walks, frog jumps, kangaroo jumps, crab walks.

Dividing:

For partners, ask the children to find a friend very quickly. For groups of four, ask the partners to join up with another couple.
To form two equal groups or teams, ask the children to find a friend, then line up with their friend behind Bobby and Anna. All the children behind Bobby become one team, and all the children behind Anna become the other team.
To form four equal groups or teams, ask the children to find a friend. Then ask them to link arms with another couple to form lines of four in front of the teacher.
These lines of four are split from front to back to form four teams.
Do not count off. It is too time consuming.

Verbalizing:

Speak clearly.
Count clearly. Be precise.
Do not talk to just one or a few children and ignore the rest.
Incite with words like "Higher! Faster!"
Excite with an enthusiastic voice.
Use "warm fuzzies" to encourage, such as:

Very good!	Much better!	Very nice.
Wonderful!	I like that.	That's different.
Super!	Well done!	Great!
Excellent!	Lovely!	All right!
Look at Jackie!	Fantastic!	Terrific!

Do not hesitate to say "No!," particularly when a child is endangering him/herself or another child.

Stand on the edge of a circle when giving instructions, rather than in the middle.

Do not ask the children if they want to do something.

Instead, say, *"Let's try...,"* *"Now Michael will...,"* *"Let's do that again."*

Do not say, *"Go to your right or your left."* Indicate the direction with a large sweep of the arm and say, *"Go this way or that way."*

Have a "magic word" for the day, such as, "Snap," "Snoop," "Pop".

The children do not move until they hear the word.

ASSESSMENT IN PHYSICAL EDUCATION

At the pre-school level, assessment will be informal observation of skill development and creative responses to challenges. Children should not be labelled failures at this early stage when the main idea is to hook them for life on "joy in movement." However, parents should be kept informed of progress in skill development in a *positive* way.

At the primary level, assessment, evaluation, and grading in physical education are often dictated by the policy of the school district. This policy may go totally against the philosophy of assessment held by the teacher; so many times a compromise will have to be made, mostly on the part of the teacher.

Agreement must be reached on the *what, why,* and *how* of assessment. Children can be assessed on:

Attainment of stated objectives.

Achievement of a certain skill level.

Skill improvement.

Skill application in a game situation.

Sportsmanship.

Rules and strategies.

Participation.

Nonparticipation without satisfactory excuse.

If some or all of the above items are selected, they must be clearly conveyed to children, parents, and school administrators before a program begins. They must be defensible, and a necessary part of the total educational program.

Teachers should use both *formative* and *summative* assessments. Formative assessment occurs early and during the semester to let the children know where they need to *improve*. Summative assessment usually occurs at the end of a unit or semester to show what the children have *achieved*. It is the latter that is most often used in grade assignment.

Health-related fitness testing should be first formative, then summative to see if personal goals have been reached and standards of performance achieved. Motor fitness tests can be formative, but are generally summative.

SAFETY

Accidents happen even in the safest environments. In an activity lesson, children are moving and taking risks; the chances of an accident occurring are much higher than when they are sitting in a classroom. Parents do not expect the impossible from teachers, but they do expect their children to be educated in a safe, well-supervised environment by sensible and competent teachers.

Rules for a Safe Environment:

Check equipment and facilities regularly.
Keep a record of these checks.
Report all hazards and defective equipment to the principal *in writing*.
Keep a dated copy of these reports.
Remove defective equipment or place out of bounds.
Do not continue to use it.
Check teaching area daily.
Have first class of the day perform an "Emu Parade."
Class lines up shoulder to shoulder at side of teaching area.
Children move slowly forward, picking up rocks, glass, litter in their line of movement.
Make a contest to see who collects the most.
Repeat the "Emu Parade" after lunch.
Define teaching area boundaries and insist that children stay within them.
Post safety signs and rules in gymnasium, and playground.
Secure a facility after use.

Prudent Teaching Strategies:

Condition children well.
Do not overextend unfit children initially.

Follow appropriate skill progressions.
Do not allow activities beyond the skill level of the children.
Do not allow unfair competition between children who are mismatched in size, strength, and skill level.
Have adequate spacing between activities to avoid collisions.
Never finish races or relays at a wall or fence.
Warn children of risks involved in certain activities.
Do not force children to attempt an activity that they indicate they do not have the skill to perform.
Make sure children wear protective equipment such as shin guards, batting helmets.
Do not attempt to teach an activity that you are not qualified to teach.
Control the class; do not allow mayhem.

Supervision Strategies:

Never leave the activity lesson unsupervised.
Never allow unsupervised use of equipment.
Keep an eye on all children at all times.
Station yourself at the activity where specific supervision is needed, but stand in a position where the whole class is in view.

Safety First:

Establish accident procedures *before* an accident occurs.
Know the school's policy on accident procedures.
File accident reports promptly.
Obtain names of witnesses.
Remember that you are not a physician.
Render life-saving first aid and immediately seek professional help.
Keep current in first aid and CPR.
Have a small first aid kit handy.
Know where there is a supply of ice.
Never move a child who appears to have suffered a neck or back injury.
Always treat a head bruise with caution.
Notify parents if child has been hit on the head, so they can look for anything unusual in the next twenty-four hours.
Never *force* a child returning from an illness or injury to participate in an activity class.
Request a medical clearance if in doubt about a malingerer.
Know the medical histories of all children.

Request a physician's report for children with health problems or handi-
capping conditions.
Encourage the school or pre-school center to offer accident insurance.
Curtail strenuous activity in hot, humid weather.
Have drinking water available before, during, and after vigorous activity.
Discontinue outdoor activities when an electrical storm is in the area.
Carry liability insurance, but don't disclose the fact to *anyone*.

Wrongful Accusation:

A relatively recent unfortunate trend is the increased number of
accusations of child molestation leveled against caregivers and teachers.
The following warnings may help to forestall wrongful accusations:

Never keep just one child after class to put away equipment.

Never keep just one child behind after an after-school activity.

Be careful in gymnastics class not to touch children's bodies in places
    where you could be accused of sexual molestation. Nowadays, it is
    common to have sessions with young children on "good" touching
    and "bad" touching.

Never invite or take children to your home.

Never take children on field trips without at least two parents present.

If wrongfully accused, seek the advice of an attorney immediately.

Do not offer any information on the matter to *anyone*.

Chapter X

PLAYGROUNDS AND EQUIPMENT

No day care center or school ever seems to have enough money to equip a playground, so the enterprising activity teacher must make do, improvise, and use traditional equipment in nontraditional ways. In this chapter, the authors offer suggestions for establishing and equipping a playground and wall markings. These can be projects for parents, physical plant staff, or teachers.

The most critical activity when planning and equipping a playground is *risk management. Foreseeability* is the key factor in risk management. That is, the ability to examine areas and equipment for possible hazards and future accidents, and to remove or reduce as many as possible. Equally important is the need to *establish* and *enforce rules* in the playground, and to have clearly understood accident procedures. A good example of foreseeability is not to allow children to wear jackets with hood or waist drawstrings which can become entangled in equipment and could cause strangulation.

When planning playgrounds, authorities must adhere to the *Individuals with Disabilities Act (1990).* Playgrounds and equipment must be accessible to children with disabilities. Wider gates, ramps with railings, firm approaches to the playground for wheelchairs, children with leg braces or crutches are essential. Several playground equipment companies have developed play sets that are accessible, challenging, and fun.

Playgrounds and equipment must be maintained on a regular basis. Caregivers and teachers must be required to make inspections daily, and often more frequently, for broken equipment and hazards such as:

protruding nails

frayed cables

jagged edges and sharp corners

broken anchors

exposed footings

loose bolts

splintering

toxic materials

electrical hazards

standing water

spiders and snakes

Hazards must be reported *in writing.* Unsafe equipment must be removed or placed out of bounds until repaired. It cannot be emphasized too strongly that caregivers and teachers must be vigilant at all times when supervising playgrounds. There should not be any blind spots; all children must be in view at all times. This includes tunnel slides; some part of a child must be visible while descending.

ESSENTIAL ELEMENTS OF A PLAYGROUND

Fence:

A fence should be at least five feet high and difficult to climb. Gates must have locks above the reach of pre-school children. This gives peace of mind to parents, caregivers and teachers; cuts down on the possibility of accidents to children pursuing balls, and reduces vandalism to equipment.

Surfaces:

A good playground should have three surfaces:

1. Grass, preferably with both flat areas for games, and slopes for children to run up and down.
2. Fall zones, under and around equipment. They should be composed of sand, pea gravel, wood chips or other resilient materials. This area must be kept loose and soft, not compacted. To be an effective cushion against falls, the fall zone should be 6–12 inches deep under and around climbing equipment, swings and seesaws. It is *not* acceptable to place sand over concrete or other hard surfaces in fall zones.
3. Hard surface, such as blacktop, for games, ball handling skill development, tricycle lanes, and a traffic safety village. This hard surface should have markings such as circles, lines, squares, ladders,

streams and animal shapes. These markings can be invaluable for organizing children and playing simple games.

Shade and/or Shelter:

Shade trees are an inviting addition to a playground. They can be used as a refuge from the sun, for climbing, or for a nice place to tell and act out stories. A covered area, or shelter, for bad weather play and activity classes is a must; for it is on such bad days that children most need to release pent-up energy.

Traffic Lanes:

Placement of equipment in a playground is important. Good traffic lanes between and around the equipment must be maintained. In free activity, children will run from one piece of equipment to another. Items poorly positioned, or placed too close, invite collisions.

Water Fountain:

Active children need easy access to drinking water, during and after play, to replenish body fluids. If fountains are not feasible, thermos flasks with push-button spigots, and paper cups should be available.

Toilet Facilities:

If a playground is to maintain high hygienic standards, then toilet facilities must be provided. A well-planned school or day care center will have access to the toilets directly from the playground to cut down on traffic in and out of the building.

Water Play Table:

A water play table should be at a pre-school child's waist level. It should be equipped with an overflow drain that will not flow on to the general play area. Props such as boats, doll clothes to wash, sponges and plastic containers should be provided.

Developmental Sand Play Area:

A sand play area should be surrounded with low, upright logs, rail-road ties; or enclosed in a large tractor tire. This will cut down on the wind carrying sand away. The area should be inspected frequently for broken glass and trash, and covered when not in use. Buckets, spades, and various plastic containers will encourage constructive activities.

Garden:

If children are to experience the joy of planting seeds and watching them grow, a garden area must be provided in a playground. It should be placed adjacent to a water supply and preferably out of the line of daily traffic. A surround of railroad ties will help in defining the area and in holding the soil within.

EQUIPMENT

Equipment should encourage children to *move, rather than be moved.* Balance beams, sloping ladders, forts, climbing units should take priority over traditional equipment such as swings, seesaws, merry-go-rounds, and spring horses, on which children sit and are moved. Choose equipment that will provide total body development, outlets for imagination, as well as fun.

Children need to develop agility, balance, flexibility, muscular strength and endurance, and cardiovascular efficiency. They need to develop upper-body strength through climbing, hanging, swinging, and inverting. They need to test their courage in ascending and descending equipment.

Equipment must be safe, sturdy, free from jagged edges or rough surfaces and toxic materials, such as paint or creosote. Recycled materials must be examined carefully from the safety aspect before being used for playground equipment. Surfaces must have a sealant. If traditional equipment such as swings, seesaws, and merry-go-rounds are included in a playground, the following precautions must be taken:

> Swings must be placed clear of walls and fences, and out of the traffic flow from one piece of equipment to another. They should be *at least* 24 inches apart and 30 inches from sturdy supports firmly anchored in concrete at least 6 inches underground. Seats should be made of soft material such as pliable plastic. Chains should not have pinch points for little fingers. Overhead hook attachments must be closed. As most swing-set injuries result from falls, it is important that the fall zone meets standard requirements. A jumping or falling child can be propelled forward several feet beyond the swing chain's length.
>
> Seesaws must be checked for crush points, pinch points and protruding bolts. The fulcrum must be enclosed.

Slides must be checked for protruding bolts and posts that can catch clothing. There should be an enclosed platform at the top large enough for children to retreat if they change their minds about sliding down. Sides should be at least 6 inches high. Resilient ground cover, 2 feet deep at the base of the slide, should be maintained. Worn areas at the base can expose hard surfaces and allow water to accumulate. Slide surfaces made of metal can become hot enough to burn a child. Plastic slides which stay cooler are now available.

Merry-go-rounds are fun for children but not worth the hazards they present. Children can be crushed or pinched by moving parts; clothing can be snagged, feet can be caught under the merry-go-round, especially when the ground below the edge wears away.

Ladder rungs must be further apart than nine inches (the size of a basketball) to reduce the risk of head-entrapment and strangulation.

Platforms, treehouses, and forts over 30 inches above the ground must be *enclosed* with guardrails to prevent children from slipping through. The structures should not be higher than the reaching height of an average pre-school child.

Trampolines are *not* recommended for playgrounds in this day and age of litigation. Inflated inner tubes and low-spring platforms can be fun to balance and jump on.

Small equipment, while not in use, should be locked away in an adjacent storage area. A record of maintenance and repairs must be kept.[1]

---

[1]For additional guidelines on playgrounds and equipment write the U.S. Consumer Product Safety Commission, Washington, D.C. 20207, and the American Society for Testing Materials, 1916 Race St., Philadelphia, PA 19103.

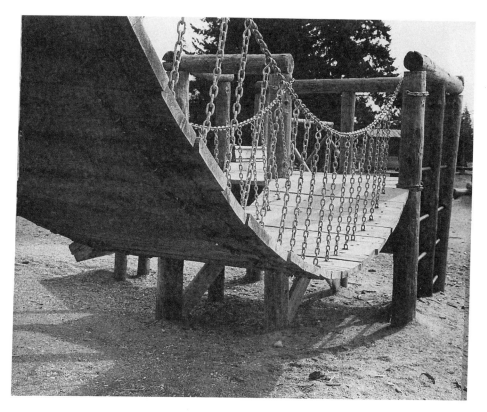

Figure 85. Adventure Playground Equipment.

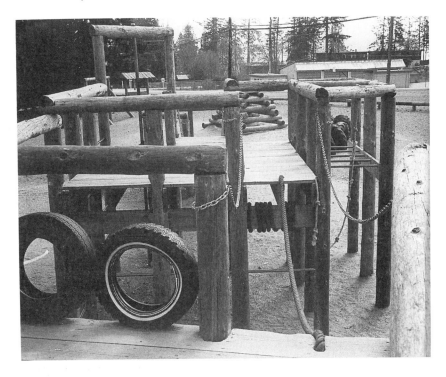

Figure 86. Adventure Playground Equipment.

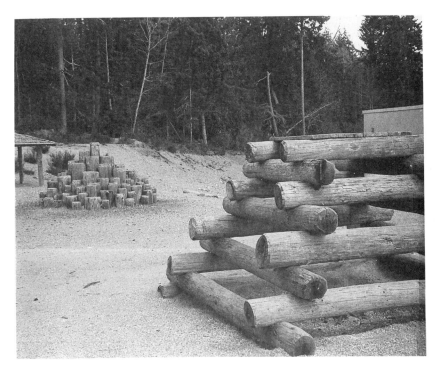

Figure 87. Adventure Playground Equipment.

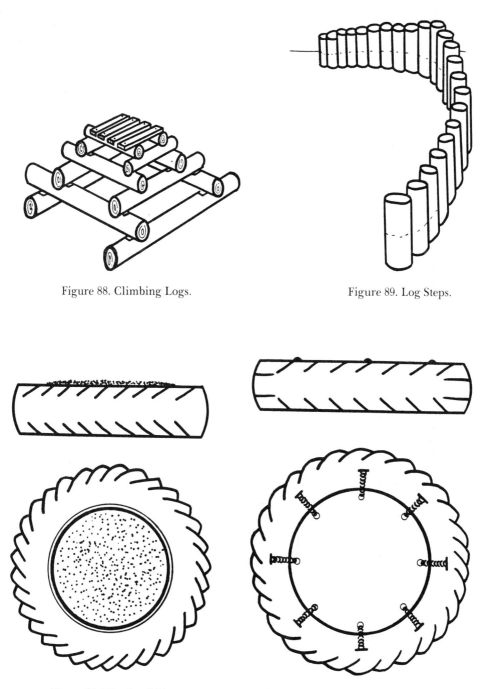

Figure 88. Climbing Logs.

Figure 89. Log Steps.

Figure 90. Tire Sand Pit.

Figure 91. Tire Mini Trampoline.

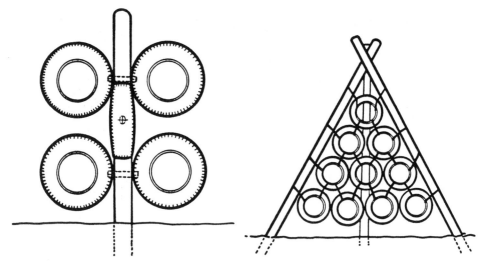

Figure 92. Tire Climbing Tree.   Figure 93. Tire Climbing Frame.

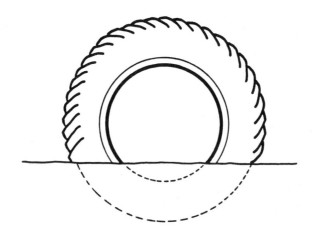

Figure 94. Tire Leap Frog/Crawl Through.

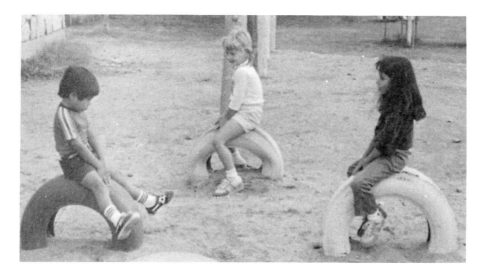

Figure 95. Tires Set in Ground. Note: Soft Playground Surface.

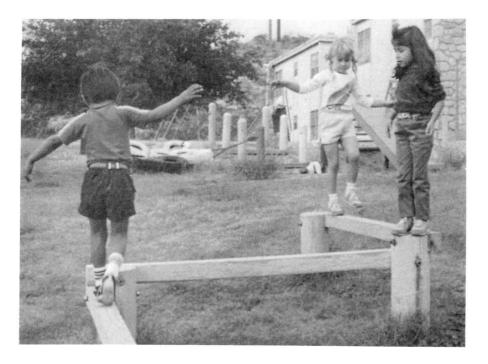

Figure 96. Balance Beam.

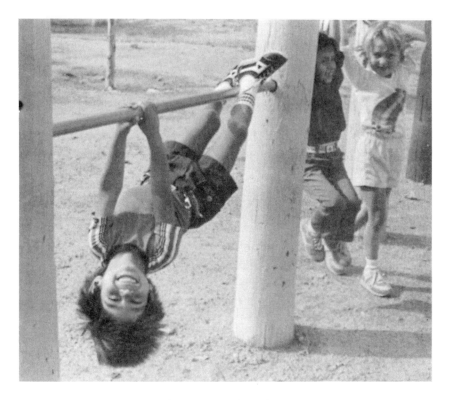

Figure 97. Horizontal Bar.

IMPROVISING EQUIPMENT

Beanbags

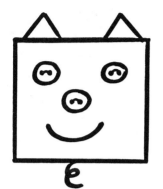

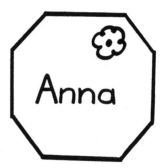

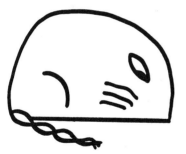

Figure 98. Beanbags: Decorated.

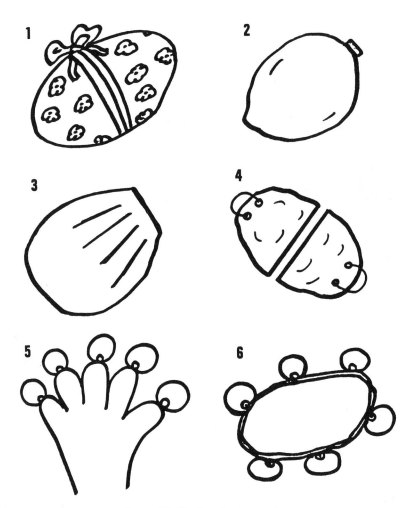

Figure 99. Rhythm Instruments.

Rhythm Instruments

1. Shaker: pantyhose container
2. Shaker: lemon juice container
3. Shaker: two large seashells
4. Castanets: walnut shells
5. Glove with bells
6. Elastic anklet with bells

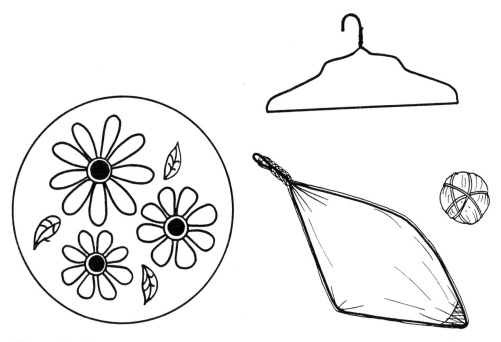

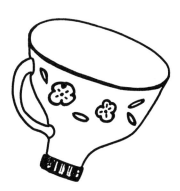

Figure 100. Frisbee: Decorated Plastic Coffee Can Lid.

Figure 101. Goodminton Racquet and Panty-hose Ball.

Figure 102. Bleach Bottle Catcher.

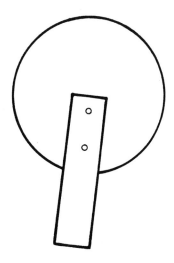

Figure 103. Wooden Paddle.

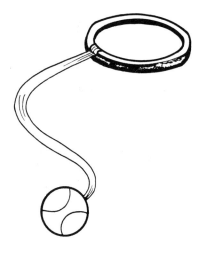

Figure 104. Plastic Ring From Bleach Bottle.

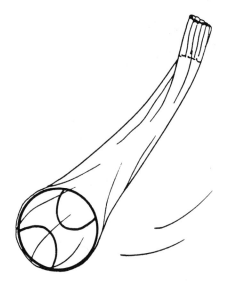

Figure 105. Handsie: Knee Hi Stocking and Ball.

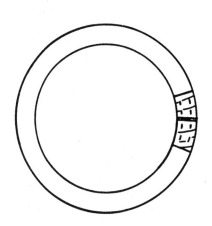

Figure 106. Plastic Hoop Made From Plumber's Pipe.

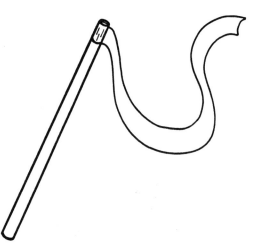

Figure 107. Crepe Paper Streamer and Stick.

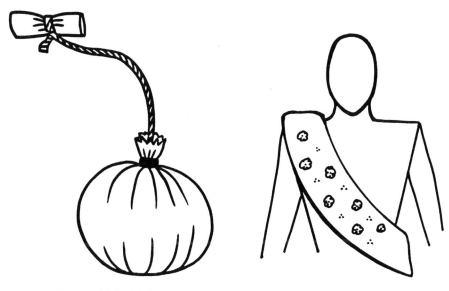

Figure 108. Poi Ball.   Figure 109. Team Band From Leftover Material.

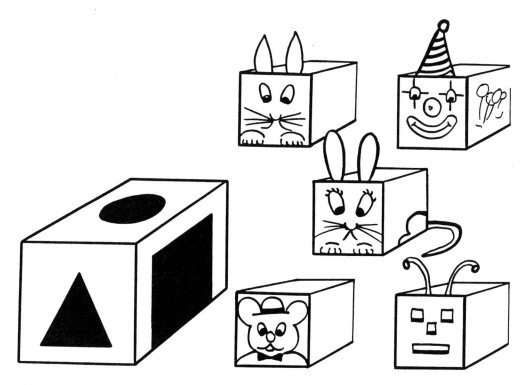

Figure 110. Target Box From Grocery Carton.   Figure 111. Boundary Markers: Decorated Cartons.

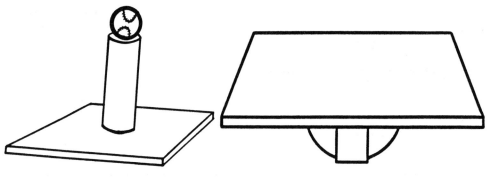

Figure 112. Batting Tee.   Figure 113. Balance Board.

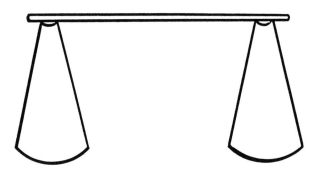

Figure 114. Hurdles: Cones and Wand.

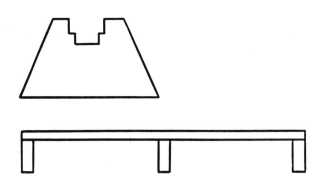

Figure 115. Low Balance Beam.

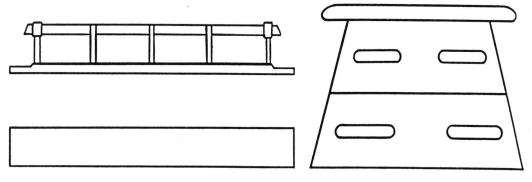

Figure 116. Bench with Balance Beam at Base.

Figure 117. Vaulting Box.

WALL MARKINGS

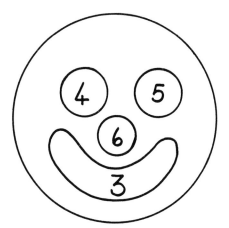

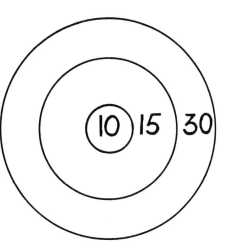

Figure 118. Wall Marking: Clown Face.

Figure 119. Wall Marking: Target.

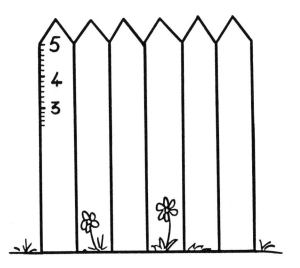

Figure 120. Wall Marking: Nosey Parker Peek Fence.

PLAYGROUND MARKINGS

Key:

1. Circles for games and dances
2. (a) and (b). Starting and finishing lines for races
3. Listening lines
4. Ladder for leaps and jumps
5. Whale for "Follow-The-Leader"
6. Stream for jumps and leaps across
7. Stepping stones for jumps, hops, leaps
8. Map for tossing beanbags from state to state; jumps, leaps, hops, "Follow-The-Leader," geography knowledge
9. Foursquare
10. Hopscotches

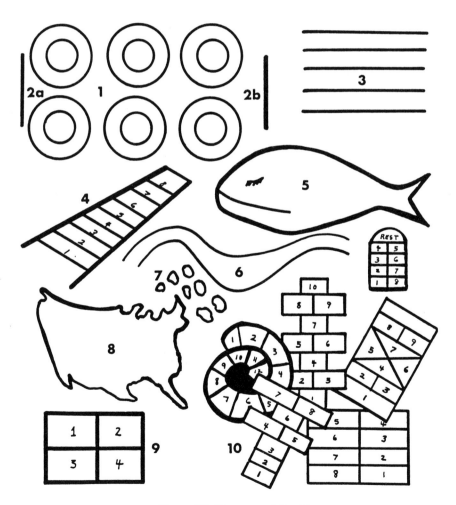

Figure 121. Playground Markings.

APPENDICES

APPENDIX A

EQUIPMENT

ABC School Supply, Inc.
3312 N. Berkeley Lake Road
Duluth, GA 30136

Adventure Playgrounds, Inc.
University of Cincinnati
College of Designs, Architecture and Art
Cincinnati, OH 45221

American Athletic
200 American Avenue
Jefferson, IA 50129

Beckley-Cardy
1 East First Street
Duluth, MN 55802

Childs/Play
P.O. Box 448
Eureka Springs, AR 72632

Cole Educational Supply
P.O. Box 34915
Houston, TX 77234

Community Playthings
P.O. Box 901
Rifton, NY 12471

Cosom/Schaper
P.O. Box 1426
Minneapolis, MN 55440

Cramer Physical Educational Supplies
P.O. Box 1001
Gardner, KS 66030

Creative Schoolhouse, Inc.
2501 West Ohio
Midland, TX 79701

Discovery Toys
313 Post Oak Drive
Lewisville, TX 75060

Educational Activities, Inc.
P.O. Box 392
Freeport, NY 11520

Elementary Gym Closet
2511 Leach Road
Auburn Heights, MI 48057

Environments, Inc.
P.O. Box 1348
Beaufort, SC 29901

Flaghouse for Special Populations
150 N. MacQuestin Parkway
Mt. Vernon, NY 10550

Bill Fritz Sports Corporation
P.O. Box 860
Cary, NC 27512

GOPHER
2929 W. Park Drive
Owatonna, MN 55060

Grounds for Play, Inc.
3501 Ave. E East
Arlington, TX 76011

Holbrook-Patterson, Inc.
Coldwater, MI 49036

Hoover Brothers, Inc.
2050 Postal Way
Dallas, TX 75212

Jayfro Corporation
P.O. Box 400
Waterford, CT 06385

Kaplan
P.O. Box 609
Lewisville, NC 27023

Kids Kubes
Iron Mountain Forge
P.O. Box 897
Farmington, MO 63640

Landscape Structures, Inc.
Route 2, Box 26
Delano, MN 55328

Nickel Industries, Inc.
1913 S. W. Freeway
Houston, TX 77098

Playworld Systems
315 Cherry Street
New Berlin, PA 17855

Quality Playground Equipment
P.O. Box 58
Tomball, TX 77377

Retro Toys
4245 N. Central Freeway
Dallas, TX 75205

Rifton for People with Disabilities
Rifton, NY 12471

Snitz Sports Supply Company
104 South Church Street
East Troy, WI 53120

Sportime
One Sportime Way
Atlanta, GA 30340

Things From Bell
P.O. Box 206
Princeton, WI 54968

Toledo Physical Education Supply, Inc.
P.O. Box 5618
Toledo, OH 43613

Wham-O, Inc.
San Gabriel, CA 91778

W. J. Voit Rubber Corporation
29 Essex Street
Maywood, NJ 07607

Wolverine Sports
Box 1941
Ann Arbor, MI 48106

APPENDIX B

MUSIC

Bowmar Music and Records
Division Belwin Mills
Melville, NY 11747

Cats Paws in Motion
9115 Cross Mountain Trail
San Antonio, TX 78255

Chime Time
2440-C Pleasantdale Road
Atlanta, GA 30340

Educational Activities, Inc.
157 Chambers Street
New York, NY 10017

Folk Dance Records
3022 South Washington Street
Seattle, WA 98144

Folkways Records
117 West Forty-sixth Street
New York, NY 10036

Hoctor Records
Waldwick, NJ 07463

Kimbo Educational Music and Movement
P.O. Box 477
Long Branch, NJ 07740

Kiwi Records
A. H. & A. W. Reed, Ltd.
Wellington, New Zealand

Leo's Advance Theatrical Company
2451 Sacramento Avenue
Chicago, IL 60647

Merrback Record Service
P.O. Box 7308
323 West 14th Street
Houston, TX 77008

Statler Records, Inc.
1795 Express Drive North
Smithtown, NY 11787

The Lloyd Shaw Foundation
Recordings Division
The Millhouse
Roxbury, NY 12474

BIBLIOGRAPHY

Aquatics

Langendorfer, Steve & Bruya, Larry (1995). *Aquatic readiness.* Champaign, IL: Human Kinetics.

YMCA (1987). *Y skippers: An aquatic program for children five and under.* Champaign, IL: Human Kinetics.

Dance

Boorman, Joyce (1969). *Creative dance in the first three grades.* New York: David McKay, Inc.

Burnett, Millie (1975). *Dance down the rain, sing up the corn.* San Francisco: R. & E. Research Associates, Inc.

Department of Education (1967). *Games and dances of the Maori.* Wellington, New Zealand: Government Printers.

Fleming, Gladys A. (Ed.). (1990). *Children's dance.* Reston, VA: AAHPERD.

Gilbert, Anne G. (1992). *Creative dance for all ages.* Reston, VA: AAHPERD.

Joyce, Mary (1984). *Teaching dance technique to children.* Palo Alto, CA: National Press.

Laban, Rudolf (1975). *Modern educational dance.* London: MacDonald and Evans.

Lloyd, Marcia (1990). *Adventures in creative movement activities: A guide to teaching.* Reston, VA: AAHPERD.

National Dance Association (1990). *Guide to creative dance for the young child.* Reston, VA: AAHPERD.

Overby, Lynnette, Y. (Ed.). (1991). *Early childhood creative arts.* Reston, VA: AAHPERD.

Purcell, Theresa M. (1994). *Teaching children dance: Becoming a master teacher.* Champaign, IL: Human Kinetics.

Russell, Joan (1975). *Creative movement and dance for children.* London: MacDonald and Evans.

Stinson, Sue (1988). *Dance for young children: Finding the magic in movement.* Reston, VA: AAHPERD.

Stinson, William (Ed.). (1990). *Moving and learning for the young child.* Reston, VA: AAHPERD.

U.N.I.C.E.F. (1967). *Hi neighbour, fun and folklore.* New York: United States Council for UNICEF.

General Physical Education and Sport

Barlin, Anne L. & Kalev, Nurit (1989). *Hello toes! Movement games for children.* Reston, VA: AAHPERD.

Buschner, Craig A. (1994). *Teaching children movement concepts and skills.* Champaign, IL: Human Kinetics.

Coquitlam School District (1992). *Elementary physical education curriculum, primary.* Coquitlam, B.C., Canada: Curriculum Department.

Department of Education (1955). *Physical education, infant division.* Wellington, New Zealand: Government Printers.

Department of Education (1967). *Physical education in junior classes.* Wellington, New Zealand: Government Printers.

Diem, Liselott (1957). *Who can?* Kassel, Germany: Meister Druck.

Diem, Liselott (1991). *The important early years.* Reston, VA: AAHPERD.

Gallahue, David (1989). *Understanding motor development: Infants, children, adolescents.* Dubuque, IA: Brown.

Graham, G., Holt/Hale, S., & Parker, M. (1993). *Children moving.* Palo Alto, CA: Mayfield.

Hammett, Carol Totsky (1992). *Movement activities for early childhood.* Champaign, IL: Human Kinetics.

Haywood, K. (1993). *Life span motor development.* Champaign, IL: Human Kinetics.

Humphrey, James H. (1992). *Motor learning in childhood education.* Springfield, IL: Charles C Thomas.

Humphrey, James H. (1994). *Physical education for the elementary school.* Springfield, IL: Charles C Thomas.

Humphrey, James H. (1994). *Sports for children: A guide for adults.* Springfield, IL: Charles C Thomas.

I.C.H.P.E.R. (1967). *Book of worldwide games and dances.* Washington, DC: NEA Publications.

Logsdon, B., et al. (1994). *Physical Education Teaching Units for Program Development, Grades K–3.* Champaign, IL: Human Kinetics.

Morrison, Ruth (1969). *A movement approach to educational gymnastics.* London: J. M. Dent.

Nichols, Beverly (1990). *Moving and learning: The elementary school physical education experience.* St. Louis: Times Mirror/Mosby.

Pangrazi, R. P. & Dauer, V. P. (1995). *Dynamic physical education for elementary school children.* Boston, MA: Allyn and Bacon.

Pica Rae (1990). *Preschoolers moving and learning.* Champaign, IL: Human Kinetics.

Pica Rae (1991). *Special themes for moving and learning.* Champaign, IL: Human Kinetics.

Riggs, M. L. (1990). *Jump to Joy.* Englewood Cliffs, NJ: Prentice-Hall.

Rink, J. (1993). *Teaching physical education for learning.* St. Louis: C. V. Mosby.

Scottish Office Education Department (1992). *Curriculum and assessment in Scotland national guidelines, expressive arts 5–14.* Edinburgh: Her Majesty's Stationery Office.

Siedentop, D. (1991). *Developing teaching skills in physical education.* Palo Alto, CA: Mayfield.

Sporting Goods Manufacturers Association (1990). *Ideas for action: Award winning approaches to physical activity.* North Palm Beach, FL: SGMA.

U.S. Department of Education (1991). *America 2000: An education strategy.* Washington, D.C.: U.S. Department of Education.

Werner, Peter H. (1994). *Teaching children gymnastics.* Champaign, IL: Human Kinetics.

Williams, J. (1987). *Themes for educational gymnastics.* London: Black.

Health and Fitness for Life

Breighner, Kathryn & Rohe, Deborah (1990). *I am amazing.* Circle Pines, MN: American Guidance Service.

Cheung, Lilian W. Y. & Richmond, Julius B. (Eds.). (1995). *Child health, nutrition, and physical activity.* Champaign, IL: Human Kinetics.

Corbin, C. B. & Lindsey, R. (1994). *Concepts of physical fitness.* Dubuque, IA: Brown/Benchmark.

Edlin, Gordon & Golanty, Eric (1992). *Health and wellness.* Boston, MA: Jones and Bartlett.

Fish, Helen T., Fish, Ronald B. & Golding, Lawrence A. (1989). *Starting out well, a parent's approach to physical activity and nutrition.* Champaign, IL: Leisure Press.

Hoeger, Werner & Hoeger, Sharon (1992). *Lifetime physical fitness and wellness.* Englewood, CO: Morton.

Humphrey, James H. (1991). *An overview of childhood fitness: Theoretical perspectives and scientific bases.* Springfield, IL: Charles C Thomas.

Humphrey, James H. (1993). *Elementary school child health: For parents and teachers.* Springfield, IL: Charles C Thomas.

Karnes, Merle B. (1992). *Fit for me.* Circle Pines, MN: American Guidance Service.

Maione, Mary Jane (1989). *Kids weigh to fitness.* Reston, VA: AAHPERD.

Pangrazi, Robert P. & Corbin, Charles B. (1994). *Teaching strategies for improving youth fitness.* Reston, VA: AAHPERD.

Page, Parker, Cieloha, Dan & Suid, Murray (1990). *Getting along.* Circle Pines, MN: American Guidance Service.

Pate, Russell & Hohn, Richard C. (Eds.) (1994). *Health and fitness through physical education.* Champaign, IL: Human Kinetics.

Rotatori, Anthony F. & Fox, Robert A. (1989). *Obesity in children and youth: Measurement, characteristics, causes and treatment.* Springfield, IL: Charles C Thomas.

Rowland, Thomas W. (1990). *Exercise and children's health.* Champaign, IL: Human Kinetics.

U.S. Department of Health and Human Services (1990). *Healthy people 2000: National health promotion and disease prevention objectives.* Washington, DC: U.S. Government Printing Office.

Play

Blanchard, Kendall (Ed.). (1986). *The many faces of play.* West Point, NY: Leisure Press.
Herron, R. E. & Sutton-Smith, B. (Eds.). (1971). *Child's play.* New York: John Wiley.
Manning, F. E. (Ed.). (1983). *The world of play.* West Point, NY: Leisure Press.
Piaget, J. (1962). *Play, dreams and imitation in childhood.* New York: Norton.
Smilanski, S. (1968). *The effects of sociodramatic play on disadvantaged preschool children.* New York: John Wiley.

Playgrounds and Safety

Bruya, Larry & Langendorfer, Steve (Eds.). (1988). *Where our children play: Elementary school playground equipment.* Reston, VA: AAHPERD.
Bruya, Larry (Ed.). (1988). *Play spaces for children: A new beginning.* Reston, VA: AAHPERD.
Della-Guistina, Daniel E. & Yost, Charles P. (1991). *Teaching safety in the elementary school.* Reston, VA: AAHPERD.
National Safety Council (1990). *Accident facts: 1990 education.* Chicago: National Safety Council.
Wortham, Sue C. & Frost, Joe L. (1990). *Playgrounds for young children: National survey and perspectives.* Reston, VA: AAHPERD.

Special Physical Education

Carter, Marcia K., Dolan, Mary A. & LeConey, Stephen P. (1994). *Designing instructional swim programs for individuals with disabilities.* Reston, VA: AAHPERD.
Grosse, Susan J. & Thompson, Donna (Eds.) (1993). *Play and recreation for individuals with disabilities: Practical pointers.* Reston, VA: AAHPERD.
Levine, Susan P., et al. (1983). *Recreation experiences for the severely impaired or nonambulatory child.* Springfield, IL: Charles C Thomas.
Morris, Lisa R. & Schulz, Linda (1989). *Creative play activities for children with disabilities.* Champaign, IL: Human Kinetics.
Raynor, Sherry & Drouillard, Richard (1978). *Get a wiggle on.* Reston, VA: AAHPERD.
Sherrill, Claudine (Ed.). (1988). *Leadership training in adapted physical education.* Champaign, IL: Human Kinetics.
Trief, Ellen (1992). *Working with visually impaired young students: A curriculum guide for birth–3 year olds.* Springfield, IL: Charles C Thomas.